Jennifer Jolan's Big Book of Diets

All You Need to Know about 50 of the World's Most Popular Diets

---

The Good, the Bad, and the Ugly!

JENNIFER JOLAN

http://WeightLossEbookStore.com

TABLE OF CONTENTS

Jennifer Jolan

ABOUT THE AUTHOR
(And Get A Free Book)

Jennifer Jolan is a best-selling author and "America's Weight Loss Queen."

Over 120,000 people have read her "How to Lose Weight Spinning Around in a Circle Like Kids" book, and thousands more have bought her best-selling "1 Day Diet" book.

In addition, she has written over 1,100 articles about weight loss, and has helped thousands of people around the world fix their weight problems without starvation, restrictive dieting, or struggle.

As a special gift for getting this book, you can get a **free** copy of Jennifer's smash hit book *How to Lose Weight Spinning Around In A Circle Like Kids* (which sells for $19.95 elsewhere) on her website at:

http://WeightLossEbookStore.com/bonus

INTRODUCTION

Diets, diets, diets, everywhere are diets!

Low-fat diets, high-fat diets, grapefruit-only diets, cottage cheese-only diets, low-carb diets, high-carb diets, no-carb diets... Arrgh! Somebody needs to put some sanity into all this. And I'm just the one to do it for you!

In this tome, I break them all down for you. I survey all the popular diets. And there're a lot of them! And to show how popular they can be, I bet you've heard of and know some about at least half of them.

How can one diet prescribe exactly the opposite of another and *both* help you lose weight? Many reasons exist as to why this is possible although there are a few that certainly are suspect and have their detractors who say that some of these popular diets add up to big failures.

- I'll try to do my best to be objective and just give you the facts on each of the diets!

- I'll tell you what is good and what is bad!

- I'll describe each one in a nutshell to remove the fog from this massive universe of diets!

- I'll tell you the problems with them, why you might want to avoid some of them like the plague, and why some are considered to be realistic and proven ways to lose weight and *keep it off!*

Many of these diets easily fall into the category of *Fad Diet* or *Crash Diet*. Many of these kinds of fad and crash diets fail miserably because they do not provide a lifetime of eating properly. Instead, they give you a short-term way to — yes — lose some weight right away... at the expense of gaining it all back *and more* later. We've all done this. You know what I mean.

The good news is that you can take pieces of many of these diets and incorporate them into your own diet and eating plan. Build one that will work *for you.* Even better, build an eating system for life so you follow a *simple* and realistic approach for maintaining your healthy weight the rest of your life. Won't that be a pleasure? It'll be easy too.

Keep an open mind and take what you can from this book's survey of 50 diets. You'll soon see that the *Big Book of Diets* is really the only book you need to learn the good and the bad of all the diets you've seen and wondered about. Obviously we cannot list every detail about every diet; if you find one or more diets you're interested in, you owe it to yourself to learn more about that diet before you decide if it's right for you.

Let's get to it.

THE 17-DAY DIET

One of the most successful diets (meaning it's sold many books) in recent history is the 17-Day Diet. The 17-Day Diet was designed by Dr. Mike Moreno.

Promising to shed pounds "safely and effectively." Does it fulfill its promise?

It's subtitled, "A Doctor's Plan." Always be skeptical! Just because something is designed by a doctor rarely makes something healthy these days. You must make sure that the doctor understands the dangers of popular food myths, is not sitting in the pharmaceutical's back pockets, and knows the proven problems with the Government's bodyfat-promoting food pyramid.

Let's see what the 17-Day diet is all about.

Overview

In its first 17 days, the 17-Day Diet promises "fast results." It states you "might" expect to lose up to 10 to 12 pounds the first 17 days. In all fairness, that "might" word is good because nobody can assure that you will always lose weight under any plan. People are too different and have too many different variables such as your starting weight and obesity level, your normal metabolism rate, and so on.

For 17 days you are restricted to certain foods. At the end of the 17 days, you switch to a different set of foods.

The Good...

By changing your diet every 17 days, your body is supposed to be "fooled" into not becoming complacent and plateauing. In addition, you don't get bored as long as you can hold out for 17-days on food groups that are next which you don't like.

The Bad and The Ugly

The book suggests that the faster you lose weight, the easier it will be to keep it off.

This certainly goes against the grain of the history of dieting! Rapid weight loss plans almost always cause their participants to gain it all back and more as you'll see throughout much of this book.

Still, you almost will find it impossible *not* to lose weight on the 17-Day Diet.

In addition, Dr. Moreno admits that your most rapid weight loss will be comprised of water and not fat. He insists that "water is weight too." That technically is sure true. But do you want to lose water or fat?

And will this diet make you lose fat *and keep it off?*

The reason so many diets fail is they are complicated. Changing everything you eat every 17 days means you often have to change the groceries you buy and the places you eat out. If you're by yourself and you don't mind the effort that is all well and good. But if you have a family you can't expect them to change their likes every 17 days to match your diet's requirements.

Note: Things can really get complicated when you begin the 17-Day Diet's requirement of alternating between two of the cycles every other day!

This being a "rapid weight loss diet" instead of a lifetime eating plan means it falls into the same category of many other diets: Failure is going to come even if one loses a lot of weight. If you cannot find an eating plan that has enough variety *and* is good for you *and* that will enable you to lose weight and keep it off, history shows that virtually *everybody* on such a diet will stop following the diet's tenants eventually.

Note: To be fair, I must tell you that the change-up every 17 days doesn't last forever. At the end of four cycles of 17-day eating plans, the 17-Day Diet puts you on an eating plan that enables you to "enjoy your favorite foods on weekends" while following a specific diet the rest of the week.

Your Big Takeaway Tip from this Diet

Variety is the spice of life and being on a diet that changes its food contents every 17 days has appeal. To many people, especially women, eating the same basic diet for long term can get monotonous. Men typically can do better on the same food for longer periods of time but everybody can get tired of the same old food.

So for variety, the 17-Day Diet is one you probably won't become bored with.

In addition, if the premise that rapid weight loss is better than slow weight loss – which again goes against the grain of every diet plan ever studied – then if true, you can find other diets that take off more with less effort. You can even try one of the starvation diets and have more rapid weight loss than the 17-Day Diet provides. (I am not recommending any starvation diet.)

Note: I'm just saying you could lose more weight faster. The problem is you'll almost certainly put it right back on and more after you finish the starvation diet.

The 17-Day Diet is better for your health than a starvation diet even if it's not as rapid in its weight loss.

THE CHINA STUDY

The China Study seems more to be a warning against certain foods than a prescription diet plan you can follow to lose weight.

Some nutritional sacred cows are thrown out too... literally! The China Study bans animal products as much as possible.

So do the Eastern countries in Asia know something we don't? Or are other factors at work?

Overview

The China Study calls itself, "The most comprehensive study on nutrition ever conducted."

Whether this is accurate or not, the results of the authors, father-and-son team T. Colin Campbell, Ph.D. and Thomas M. Campbell II, M.D. sure warn against the use of animal products in your diet. The results of the China Study seem to indicate that a vegan plant food diet reduces the chances of early mortality rates as opposed to diet with animal products which their results are said to correlate with obesity, coronary heart disease, osteoporosis, and more.

The Good...

Any eating plan that is proven to reduce major health problems needs to be looked at more closely.

Can you almost be assured that you'll have no major health problems by eating a proper diet? If yes, almost every creator of every diet in this book will agree with that. So it makes sense that we analyze foods that might cause health problems in the long term.

The Bad and The Ugly

The problem here though is that cause and effect is not easily proved. If eliminating animal products from a diet and going vegan eliminates most health problems including cancer and heart disease, then how can one explain the Inuits?

A major study of the native Inuits showed that generation after generation eating virtually nothing but seal blubber and fish and had an exceedingly low occurrence of heart and cancer problems.

The Inuits (Eskimo-like people) studies certainly *seem to* violate every tenant of the China Study.

Seeming to violate does *not* inviolate the China Study necessarily. It just shows that cause and effect are not easy to correlate to health problems. If that were simple, all of us who want to be healthy would eat exactly the same thing.

Although the Asians studied who lived a vegan lifestyle had less cancer and heart issues than the typical Westerners have, it *could not have been the vegan diet that kept those diseases away since the Inuits ate almost 100% animal protein and fat with a similar lack of cancer and heart disease as the vegan Asians studied.*

Two directly opposing results cannot both be correct. Either only one is correct, they both are wrong, or other factors came into play that were ignored intentionally or omitted by ignorance.

I'll get back to cause and effect in a moment but just use your eyes: How many people who have been vegans for several years do you know actually look healthy?

Yea, not many. That is the problem with cause and effect though. Do people become vegans because they are thin and lanky and unhealthy which is why so many look bad, or do they start looking bad because they've been vegans for several years and their resulting bodies are due to the poor nutrition?

The Inuits did eventually begin to show signs of disease. The interesting thing is *when* they began to show disease. The Inuits had virtually no breast cancer, heart disease, or high cholesterol *until* they became more westernized. This means that they began eating grains, fruits, and vegetables and slowly began getting sicker as a whole. As they progressed economically and began assimilating more into the Western culture they branched out into more processed foods in addition to the added vegetables and fruits in their diets.

Also, other factors might have limited and reduced diseases other than the type of food the Asians ate. Instead of praising a vegan diet, perhaps one should blame the origins of the food the non-Asians ate.

As food becomes more processed, whether vegetables or animal products, and as food producers use more and more fertilizers and hormones, and as animals are raised in 2x3 foot pens their whole lives and fed nothing but hormone-injected, antibiotic-laden corn meal (corn is a grain, not a vegetable like grass, and yet cow bodies are designed to eat grass and roam free), then the resulting cattle's meat becomes something changed from its natural state. And the health of the *eaters* of those animals can only be affected by such changes from the natural state of the meat.

Note: Eggs and milk have the same problems. If you don't eat hormone-free, cage-free eggs or raw, whole milk, you are perhaps harming yourself and your family. Dr. William

Campbell Douglass (*The Raw Truth About Milk*) proves conclusively how dangerous, for example, pasteurized, homogenized milk is to our bodies. The milk is not the problem, it is the *process* of the milk that is the problem.

Your Big Takeaway Tip from this Diet

There is absolutely *no way* that a vegan diet can be the reason that Asians showed less disease over the more meat-intensive West if the meat- and animal-fat-only Inuits also showed a lack of such diseases when they ate virtually no vegetables whatsoever their entire lives.

Instead of focusing on the actual foods you eat, you should focus on the *source of those foods*. No study has ever shown that raw milk is bad for you or that grass-fed beef is bad for you or that mercury-free wild Alaskan salmon is bad for you. Quite the opposite.

If you hate the taste of meat, don't eat meat. But if you like meat make sure you eat well-sourced meat that you know the origins of. Enjoy that steak, or heck, enjoy as much seal blubber as you like, as long as you know the animal was not pen-raised with hormones and antibiotics given from birth and fed nothing but corn.

THE SONOMA DIET

Variety is the spice of life!

And variety of our food is a special kind of variety we all usually enjoy most. The Sonoma Diet promises variety in that we can eat a wide assortment of food and still lose weight.

Sounds good, where do I sign up?

Overview

Dr. Connie Guttersen, Ph.D. created the Sonoma Diet in an effort to get those who fail on other diets to have a chance at losing weight. The advantage of the Sonoma Diet is the wide variety of food you're allowed to eat.

Although this might also be its downfall as you'll see... Still, variety is certainly something that sounds good and that appeals to many of us.

The Sonoma Diet starts off being a fairly strict diet but lets you loosen up as you lose pounds, eventually letting you eat sugar without guilt. The idea is to take what you eat in moderation. Enjoy what you eat, just don't eat too much of it. Nuts, fish, fruits, and vegetables are allowed.

The Good...

The suggested meat in this varied diet is fish. Fish is extremely healthy as long as you avoid the mercury-filled fish that comes in most cans, restaurants, and food sections and stick with the low mercury such as wild Alaskan Salmon.

The Sonoma diet is not a rapid weight loss diet. That is generally good except for the morbidly obese folks who need to get some poundage off immediately. The fruit and grains in the Sonoma Diet ensure that you don't lose too rapidly.

The Bad and The Ugly

In spite of the variety of foods promoted, the sad part of the Sonoma Diet is that whole grains are also part of the plan but not much beef or chicken. Your body really wasn't designed to handle grains of any kind.

Grass-fed beef and free-range chicken and eggs are an important source of nutrients. The egg has been called "the perfect food" by many food experts. In addition, low-fat dairy products are suggested for the early part of the Sonoma Diet.

Low-fat anything will ensure you don't lose as much weight as you otherwise would. Did you know they feed skim milk to calves to *fatten them up?* Quality animal or dairy fat does *not* make you fat. Quite the opposite actually and sticking with low-fat helps slow down weight loss.

Your Big Takeaway Tip from this Diet

Given that carbs equal bigger thighs, any food variety that includes them requires that you eat in moderation. When it comes to starchy and virtually fiberless carbs (such as potatoes and pasta) you need to reduce your intake of those dramatically to see a prolonged weight loss and you need to stay off those foods to keep the weight off.

Given that it's the reduction in these carb quantities that probably contribute the most to the Sonoma Diet, you might want to short-circuit the time required to lose weight and skip the Sonoma Diet and focus on one that concentrates more fully on eliminating the bad carbs altogether.

Still, if you're hungry and find yourself needing a change for a while, not dramatic weight loss, the Sonoma diet is not a horrible diet to be on and its restrictions, while not offering rapid weight loss, do provide moderate weight loss eventually. And slow and steady weight loss is certainly the rate most dieticians agree is best for a good, long-term healthy weight.

EAT RIGHT FOR YOUR TYPE
(OR THE BLOOD TYPE DIET)

Does your blood determine what you can eat?

The proponents of the Blood Type Diet (also called the Eat Right for Your Type diet) say yes.

Do you even *know* your blood type? Most people don't.

Overview

The Blood Type Diet says that your blood type determines what you can eat. If you match your specific diet to your blood type's needs, you will lose weight, be healthier, live longer, grow taller, be funnier, and make more money. (Actually, I made up some of those things.)

Primarily, Peter D'Adamo designed the Blood Type Diet and promoted it in his book, *Eat Right 4 Your Type*.

D'Adamo promotes the following eating plans for these four blood types:

- Type O – High protein diet

- Type A – Heavily vegetarian slanted with no red meat

- Type B – Dairy product heavy

- Type AB – You get to eat sort of a half-vegetarian/half dairy diet.

The Good

The Blood Type Diet sounds really scientific. That is why many have tried it. It involves blood testing of course if you don't know your blood type. That is step one before you can go further obviously.

Note: Keep in mind, a diet such as the hGC Diet sounds scientific also... it involves a medical professional injecting you with a hormone. Don't let the technical sound of something determine whether you think it's true or not.

If your blood type *does* determine how certain foods affect you then knowing your blood type and its characteristics would certainly be useful in determining your eating plan.

The Bad and The Ugly

The biggest problem is the debunked basis on which the Blood Type Diet was first based.

The Blood Type Diet is based on the *theory* of evolution. Whether you agree or disagree with evolution's factual status, nobody can disagree that the theory of evolution seems to change over time.

How it affects the Blood Type Diet is this: D'Adamo bases his various blood type eating plans on the estimated age of the four blood types. When D'Adamo first developed the Blood Type Diet, he thought Type O was the oldest so he made that a heavy meat and protein diet. His thought was that the cavemen ate mostly what they could kill and that kind of diet was best for them.

Subsequent research shows that the blood type A is older than O. Given the direct opposite approach on the eating plans between A and O, knowing which is oldest certainly dramatically shifts whether the Blood Type Diet works or is simply based on a fantasy guess at the age of blood types.

If the problem of determining the historic age of blood types was the only problem, it would still be a massive problem given how opposite the A and O diets are with the age conflict. Plus, will subsequent research prove that yet another blood type is older than either A or O?

Any of that can happen given the blood type age problem that D'Adamo has already faced.

And the blood age problem doesn't address the numerous complaints from the medical world about D'Adamo's assumptions of blood type reactions to food.

Your Big Takeaway Tip from this Diet

Given the problems of the Blood Type Diet, why not avoid it and find a more sensible solution if possible?

THE CARBOHYDRATE ADDICT'S DIET

The Carbohydrate Addict's Diet sure sounds ominous!

To me, hallucinogenic thoughts of detoxing strapped to a bed in a padded cell come to mind... but I admit that *is* a little extreme!

Actually, many people are addicted to carbohydrates in some way. Too many of the wrong carbs put too many of the wrong pounds in the wrong places. So anything to help ease our desire for carbs might be good to know about!

The Carbohydrate Addict's Diet was designed by Richard and Racher Heller, both medical doctors almost twenty years ago. Their premise is that an overeating of carbs spikes insulin levels. This produces all sorts of problems including an extra desire for more carbs.

Overview

As with Atkins, the Carbohydrate Addict's Diet severely limits your intake of carbohydrates for about 15 days. Your diet is specific and you must stick to lean meats, fish, animal fats, good oils such as essential fatty acids, and green and other richly colored vegetables. The goal is to get a lot of protein in you to curb your appetite.

Eventually you are allowed one reward meal at dinner where you can eat anything you want as long as you spend no more than one hour eating. (Long romantic dinners in Rome are out!)

The Good...

There is little room for argument: cut carbs and you will lose some weight. The amount you lose depends on how much you cut the carbs.

Note: When I discuss carbs negatively, I'm talking primarily about starchy carbs such as potatoes. And sugar-based carbs such as desserts and fructose-heavy fruit and fruit juices also count as bad carbs on almost any diet like the Carbohydrate Addict's Diet.

The Carbohydrate Addict's Diet actually allows some "low carb" desserts if you need them.

The Bad and The Ugly

As many on Atkins have found out, once you begin cheating on low-carb versions of otherwise unhealthy foods, you begin to develop once again a taste for carbs such as rich desserts. The Atkins bars and other products designed for low-carb diets seem to promote a "cheat" state-of-mind where people overdo those "legal" cheats up to the point of doing damage once again to their waistline.

But such cheat desserts really pale in comparison to eating one meal a day where you get to gobble up as much as you want within an hour!

It's true that you are more likely to stick to the Carbohydrate Addict's Diet with that evening cheat meal but you also need to understand that your weight loss is going to be agonizingly slow as you drop some pounds due to that nightly meal.

Your Big Takeaway Tip from this Diet

The basis for the Carbohydrate Addict's Diet is sound: eating protein-rich foods and healthy oils while curbing the carbs is a proven way to lose weight in a healthy manner. So many more low-carb diets, however, while being stricter than the Carbohydrate Addict's Diet, certainly are better recipes for weight loss at a more reasonable speed (meaning faster than the Carbohydrate Addict's Diet but not too fast).

THE BIGGEST LOSER CLUB

Who wants to be in the club? All of us if it means we've lost a lot of weight, right?

Playing on the television show's name, the Biggest Loser Club was created for the TV show.

Overview

The stated goal seems familiar (almost every diet in this book is touted as such!): eat healthy, lose weight, and live a healthy lifestyle that includes specific exercises.

The Good...

Unlike most dietary eating plans I outline in this book, the Biggest Loser Club has an exercise component that is a big part of the program.

The foundation of the Biggest Loser Club is calorie limitation. The "healthy eating" consists of 6 meals a day, planned for you as three "meals" and three "snacks." In general, it's agreed that multiple smaller meals are better for you than fewer large meals so this is a sound approach to tackling weight problems.

The meals all contain protein of some kind along with carbs that include grains and sauces. You can end your evening meal with fruit. We can debate the danger of spiking your fructose so close to bedtime but one piece of fruit, especially if it's organic and a low-glycemic fruit such as blueberries isn't a huge problem here.

As you can see your mealtime is varied although you must follow a rigid structure of a certain number of proteins and carb dishes at each meal and snack.

The exercises consist of a general combination of strength training (weight-bearing exercises) and cardio work. The exercises are to be done in about 30 minutes a day each day.

The Bad and The Ugly

Don't judge your probable results by the TV show of the same name! Those contestants worked out three or so hours a day at times — not 30 minutes! Do you have three hours to work out? Will you do that if you had the time?

I'm a fitness fanatic and trainer of many others but I would *never* spend three hours a day exercising. Although I am considered fit and slim already, even if I was not I know that life is too short, children grow up too fast, and the bills need to be paid. Plus the additional benefit of such prolonged exercise over that of shorter and less frequent programs isn't worth what extremely little gain I might get in those three hours.

To be fair, the Biggest Loser doesn't say you should exercise three hours a day but only 30 minutes. Still, their tie-in to the TV show sets expectations that simply cannot be met by the actual diet.

Exercise has a far less impact on your weight than the quality or quantity of food you eat. Certainly, though, if you can exercise three hours each day, the exercise is going to speed up your weight loss. Also, any muscle you build will ramp up your metabolism to help keep pounds off later.

But if you're not going to exercise as much as you might if you were on national television, you might want to skip this diet which is little more than calorie-restriction.

Your Big Takeaway Tip from this Diet

As with any calorie-limitation diet, the Biggest Loser Club sets up many for failure as soon as hunger pains kick in... and hunger pains *always* kick in. The variety of this diet, including the use of grains, causes it somewhat to be a fat-producing eating plan. The limit on the calories works only because you're actually being limited on the carbs you eat.

The exercise portion of the Biggest Loser Club will help you get toned and turn some flesh into muscle but in general the food you eat impacts your weight far more than any exercise you do.

THE NO SUGAR, NO FLOUR DIET

The No Sugar, No Flour Diet (also called the No Flour, No Sugar Diet) piqued my interest. Sugar and bread are more in the news than ever before, not as something good but as something unexpectedly worse than we ever imagined!

Scared yet?

Overview

Eat anything you want! Oh, as long as there's no sugar and no flour in it!

That is the basis of the No Sugar, No Flour Diet and its simplicity does help make it easier to follow.

The Good...

Recent studies prove conclusively how dangerous sugar is for us and how many health problems that we didn't originally attribute to sugar actually are caused by our sweet tooth.

In addition, gluten which is a special protein flour in bread that gives bread its elasticity, is now seen to cause a tremendous amount of allergy problems that we never suspected before. The more processed the flour the worse it gets. And the huge percentage of flour we eat (remember you can get flour in pizza dough, breaded entrees, and other foods you don't think of as "bread") is processed to the hilt.

Note: Bread that we've been taught to be healthy, alas, often isn't. That loaf of whole-wheat bread you get from Whole Foods still has flour. It's off-limits just as much as the white Wonder Bread.

We digest carbs quickly and we digest proteins slowly. The worse the carb (think candy bar!) the faster our bodies process it. That means we get hungry faster too. So not only do sugar and flour carbs produce more flab on our slabs but we also want more food sooner than if we ate slower-digesting more traditional protein. With protein we feel fuller longer which curbs our cravings.

The Bad and The Ugly

In spite of cutting out what might be the worse of the carbs: sugar and flour, the No Sugar, No Flour Diet is not a low-carb diet. Grains such as corn are allowed. So is tofu and other soy products that are not fermented (such as soy sauce and soy-based wine) which is thought to cause havoc with everyone's hormonal balance.

The primary plan of the No Sugar, No Flour Diet is to eliminate the worst of the carbs. This puts the diet into the calorie-limitation diet and not the low-carb dietary category.

Your weight loss will be slower than it otherwise would be and your intake of unhealthy grains such as corn could very well cause other problems down the road depending on the quantity you consume.

Your Big Takeaway Tip from this Diet

As with any calorie-limitation diet, the No Sugar, No Flour Diet will show weight loss but is also prone to cause you to stumble later when your full feeling doesn't last as long as it should.

THE SOUTH BEACH DIET

Probably no other diet sounds as sexy as the South Beach Diet!

Plus the book and magazine covers just make you want to hop on the next plane to Miami and live in the sun and tropical paradise along with all the other super-thin and healthy people!

Overview

One of the most popular diets in history is the South Beach Diet.

It's touted both as a healthy heart diet as well as a weight-loss diet.

When you read the South Beach Diet books you'll get all sorts of plans and food combinations but you can boil the South Beach Diet down to a simple low-carb eating plan. You are allowed to eat a wide variety of foods as long as you keep the high glycemic foods out of reach and out of mouth.

The Good...

The variety is the key to its popularity. People stay on the South Beach Diet for quite some time on the average as opposed to many other diets I've written about in this book.

The diet is two-phased and like many low-carb diets the first few weeks is a severely-limited carbohydrate phase where you lose some initial poundage and your body begins to get weaned off the starchy carbs to set you up for phase 2.

The goal of phase two is to add some carbs back into your diet so that you don't tire of the South Beach Diet and quit before your goals are reached.

The Bad and The Ugly

The strict eating your first two weeks or so in the first phase is difficult. If you've done Atkins you've dealt with this same preliminary carb-restricted period. Everything you eat is basically a protein with perhaps some green leafy veggies tossed in.

Another drawback is you must eat meats such as chicken without the skin, white meat preferred, and you are to stick to low-fat dairy such as cheese. The lack of fat in those foods will slow down your weight loss as I've shown elsewhere. The attack on dark meat and chicken skin has proved to put a dampening effect on many who would otherwise lose weight slightly faster and in a healthier manner at the same time. The faster weight loss if you don't cut out good fats is not going to speed up your weight loss to a level of being too rapid; quite the opposite your weight loss will be done at a more natural speed which fortunately will be faster.

Your Big Takeaway Tip from this Diet

Once you get to your ideal weight, you can monitor the South Beach Diet and stay on the diet for life if you'd like. The variety of foods might make that possible. The carbs allowed in the second phase doesn't make the South Beach Diet as rapid of a weight loss diet as many low-carb diets can do but it's thought that if you lose weight slowly but surely you are more likely to keep it off and notice the effects of the diet less.

THE ROSEDALE DIET

For diabetics and the obese, the Rosedale Diet is an extreme diet that such people might find helpful when other diets fail. The entire diet centers around the hunger hormone.

Overview

Leptin is a hormone that controls hunger. Obese and extreme diabetic patients need to destroy their hunger cravings quickly before their problems escalate into severe problems that cannot be reversed.

By controlling the hormone leptin the Rosedale Diet keeps you feeling full for longer to keep you away from the foods that put you into the position you might find yourself in.

The Good...

For quick and severe control of hunger, an immediate adherence to the Rosedale Diet is suggested for extreme cases such as the obese and diabetic.

The diet requires a consumption of healthy fats. Added protein and fats will trigger your leptin quickly.

Carbohydrates are almost non-existent on the Rosedale Diet. Carbs from green, leafy vegetables are allowed.

The Bad and The Ugly

The low allowance of proteins is a big problem. If you are on the Rosedale Diet and exercising too, you might find that the lack of protein keeps lean muscle mass from forming as quickly as it might otherwise form.

Your Big Takeaway Tip from this Diet

The lack of balance of the Rosedale Diet causes it to have problems and failures. Still, if you find yourself in an extreme state that requires an instant pouncing of your hunger, losing your first several pounds on the Rosedale Diet might be what you need to get started. Its complete lack of grains and carbs, especially for the first few weeks, keeps those danger foods away which will help you move to a more protein-rich diet after you've found success on the Rosedale Diet.

THE WEIGHT LOSS CURE

For about 60 years the Weight Loss Cure has been around but mostly forgotten until Kevin Trudeau discovered it again and brought it to the forefront of the dietary debating arena.

Want to lose a pound a day? Don't we all! The Weight Loss Cure says you will. That's quite a promise!

Overview

Instead of focusing on carbs or exercise or calories, the Weight Loss Cure focuses on cleansing your body. You must adhere to the various phases of the Weight Loss Cure if you expect to see anything like the results promised.

You are to drink a lot of water, stick to organic foods, eat a huge breakfast, and not eat past 6:00 pm.

On the second phase of the Weight Loss Cure, you're to start losing not only by following the eating plan and schedule but also by getting hGC injections. Ouch!

The Good...

The organic intake of your meals is never something I'd argue with. Today's pesticide-laden foods and hormone-injected meats and dairy might be doing nothing but killing us all off in the long run.

A big breakfast is going to satisfy an initial hunger although you'll certainly wake up much hungrier on the Weight Loss Cure than you would on any other eating plan that lets you eat past 6:00 pm.

The Bad and The Ugly

I discuss (and cuss) the use of hGC hormone injections elsewhere in this book when I discuss the hGC Hormone Diet. I will reserve most of the hormone injection discussion for that part of this book. But I will give you a preview... I don't like the idea of hormone injections for weight loss!

Let me talk about more specific arguments against the Weight Loss Cure here. One pertains to the prohibition of not being allowed to eat after 6:00 pm.

Often when people wake up in the middle of the night and can't go back to sleep, the problem is related to a lack of fat still in the digestion phase; in other words, they get hungry!

Not eating after 6:00 pm could easily turn your sleeping nights into sleepless ones so you may want to grab the bottle of Melatonin. The proponents of the Weight Loss Cure would never want you to resort to sleeping drugs such as Ambien (neither would I) given their adherence to a natural and organic detox plan to lose weight.

Many people agree that not eating close to bed time is wise. Those late calories, especially if carbohydrate-intense, will not have a chance to be worked off by your routine daily activities than if you ate them earlier in the day. There is some controversy about eating late however that you should know about.

What happens after you eat a huge meal? You get sleepy, right?

What happens there is your body is telling you that it has to digest a lot of food. Digestion is one of the most active things your body does and it takes a lot of energy to do so. To conserve enough energy to digest properly, your body promptly tries to slow you down which is why you get that sleepy feeling after a big lunch.

This is not a bad thing. By slowing down and giving your energy over to your digestion, your body can more properly absorb the food. That is why taking coffee as a pick-me-up if you get the afternoon "sleepies" isn't doing your body any favors. You're simply adding fuel to your fire allowing the non-digestive parts of your body to take over some of the energy needed elsewhere.

Some who understand the nature of digestion actually have been saying recently that eating your biggest meal at night is actually the *best* time to eat it! Yes, this goes against all you've heard but using your body's energy stores and digestion as their argument makes some sense. You generally slow down greatly after a big, nighttime meal so you give over extra energy to your digestion. The thought is, your body can digest your food better, absorb more nutrients, and general handle all that food best when you are slowing down and even going to bed to sleep.

If everything were known with certainty by everybody, then we wouldn't need so many diets! There is room for disagreement as long as objective standards are used for testing the findings of various dietary theories. Still, the digestive energy argument that supports a big, late night meal does make some sense. Plus, European countries are notorious for eating huge, multi-course meals as their last meals of the day. And in general they are leaner than Americans who don't as a culture always make the last meal of the day a gigantic pigfest.

Your Big Takeaway Tip from this Diet

Stay away from any "diet" that promotes hormone injections!

If your doctor tells you that you need such injections for any reason, first get a second opinion! If they both agree, then you may need to follow their advice or get new doctors. But don't volunteer for those.

With so many other options available, stay away from the Weight Loss Cure until further notice!

THE OATMEAL DIET

I don't really have anything against the Quakers... for example, I like their oatmeal!

And if you do too you'll love the Oatmeal Diet. I don't want to spoil things for you too early but I'll let you in on a secret: the Oatmeal Diet relies *heavily* on oatmeal! Very heavily indeed.

Overview

The Oatmeal Diet isn't a diet!

It's actually an eating regimen that involves eating lots and lots of oatmeal.

The Oatmeal Diet is *not* an actual diet. Also many variations of the Oatmeal Diet exist so you will want to peruse the literature, bookshelves, and websites for to see which variation might suit you best.

By putting oatmeal into every meal, especially and always big-time into your first meal of the day, you load up on fiber and feel full. Almost all its variants require that you include oatmeal in every meal you eat. This maintains that full feeling and keeps you packed with fiber.

The Good...

Although new research is actually beginning to question the addition of heavy fiber in our diets, most agree that we need fiber for good digestion. You certainly get fiber on the Oatmeal Diet.

Obviously you don't want to add a bunch of sugar and milk, especially low-fat, homogenized, pasteurized milk to your oatmeal. If you make organic kefir, you can eat your oats with it or perhaps with homemade yogurt to get loads of probiotics along with your oatmeal throughout the day.

The Bad and The Ugly

With this high of a high-fiber diet you're going to feel full. But in reality, you'll probably be bloated and feel exactly that way. But bloating does keep you from wanting to eat more, that's for sure.

But the Oatmeal Diet is short on protein from animal and dairy sources. You are going to lack a lot of nutrients that animal sources provide. In addition, most variations of the Oatmeal Diet comes close to a vegan diet which – much to the chagrin of vegans – can make your muscles weak and slow down any recovery from illness or broken bones.

When a diet promotes one food heavily over all the rest, I certainly shy away from it. Variety is the spice of life. While diets such as the Oatmeal Diet are simple, their drawbacks often aren't worth the benefits.

If you do go on the Oatmeal Diet for a while, be sure and grab a good, high-quality source of vitamins and minerals. This means, yes, an expensive source because such liquid nutrients often are costly if they are known to be good (and organic).

Note: A liquid nutrient is organic not just because it comes from natural sources that have not been tainted with pesticides but also because they are carbon-bound. Look for "carbon-bound" liquid nutrients if you want the vitamins and minerals that work best for your body.

Your Big Takeaway Tip from this Diet

If you insist on eating grains and increasing your fiber, you could do worse than oatmeal. (For example, you could eat corn!)

But before grabbing that big tub of oats or (worse!) a packet of instant oats, consider buying a bucket of organic *oat groats*. You can get these at Walton Feed (http://www.waltonfeed.com).

Next, get a flaker which is an attachment for a meal grinder and grind a fresh cup of oats before you eat them. This way you get the nutritional benefits of oatmeal. The nutrient loss of oatmeal after it's been flaked already is rapid. By the time it gets packed in containers and shipped to your local store, the oatmeal still has its fiber but hardly any nutrition.

Better yet, enjoy your fresh-ground oatmeal as a treat once in a while instead of making it your primary source of food by going on the Oatmeal Diet. That way you don't get so many problems from the heavy-grain and carb diet and you can enjoy a *nutritious* bowl of oatmeal as a treat every once in a while.

THE RICE DIET

Here we go...

Another diet that focuses on one specific food. You'll find several popular ones in this book that are based on a single food.

I don't hate all of them!

But if you were to ask me for a short list of foods you probably should never eat again, that short list would include potatoes, corn, and... rice!

I know what you're thinking... Asian people are generally skinny and they eat a lot of rice. Read on.

Overview

The Rice Diet in one variation or another is about 80 years old. That's been around a while, hasn't it?

The Rice Diet was developed as a relief and even promoted as a cure for kidney and hypertension diseases. After implementing this "cure" for a while the promoters saw that weight loss also occurred in patients.

The bottom line is this: Eat anything you want as long as you also eat rice. The restrictions on the non-rice foods are heavy: no sugar (so far so good if it wasn't for the rice), no processed foods (still good), no salt, and no fat.

The Good...

If you can lose weight *and* cure hypertension and kidney disorders, then why not?

Depending on your level of problem with hypertension, kidney disease, or both, if you're convinced or if your doctor is convinced that the Rice Diet will help your problems by all means it's worth trying to see if the Rice Diet reduces your symptoms or even cures your disease. In spite of some rather severe shortcomings of the Rice Diet, getting a handle on hypertension and kidney problems is worth a tremendous effort.

And attacking such problems if you can do so without medicine is a major plus.

The Bad and The Ugly

The lack of fat in your diet may very well be a problem. Your body needs an intake of healthy oils and fats (think nuts, fish oil, essential fatty acids) to function properly and to "lube your joints."

In addition opponents of the Rice Diet say most of the weight you lose will be water and not actual pounds. In addition, the heavy use of grains is not something your body was developed to handle well over time.

Your Big Takeaway Tip from this Diet

If you have kidney or hypertension problems by all means give the Rice Diet a try. You will probably lose some weight and hopefully you'll lose the health problems.

If that happens you may want to then switch to an eating plan that you can stick to for life.

THE CABBAGE SOUP DIET

Cabbage is good for you! You won't find me arguing that.

Cabbage is a rich source of nutrients and its lack of starchy carbs means that you can eat about all you want and it will never affect your scales the next morning.

Plus, you should be eating cabbage in fermented form daily if you can. It's called *sauerkraut* you know. And sauerkraut has a tremendous amount of probiotic qualities. Fix your gut and you'll fix many other health problems while keeping potential problems away.

(And I love cabbage but guess what? I hate sauerkraut! But I am getting used to it after all these years and I love the benefits it gives me. I've even started making my own sauerkraut... it's so easy to do! Unlike the store-bought sauerkraut, when you make your own you don't use heat so you keep as many of the cabbage nutrients intact as possible.)

So you'll find me eating cabbage in many forms. And Cabbage Soup?

Cabbage Soup sounds good to me... I think I'll make some tonight!

But the Cabbage Soup Diet? Ugh, I don't think so.

Overview

The Cabbage Soup Diet is simple and fortunately doesn't require anything severe like some of those extra weird diets (such as daily injections of hormones like the hGC Diet requires!)

Here's what you do: Eat a bowl of cabbage soup before meals.

Huh.

The Good

What could be simpler? And I *love* simple because we're more likely to stick with something that is simple.

The problem is that it's *not really* that simple but that is how it is often introduced. Once you learn more about it you quickly see that the Cabbage Soup Diet requires a specific set of foods eaten after your cabbage soup and you must eat this specific food on a schedule so as not to overlap the required foods from one day to the other.

Cabbage is healthy! Cabbage is loaded with vitamins and tastes good.

The Bad and The Ugly

The Cabbage Soup Diet is *loaded* with starchy carbs that include foods such as:

- Unlimited fruit on one day (except for bananas)

- Eight bananas one day (but no other fruit!)

- Potatoes and rice on one day a week and it must be at the *end* of the 7-day period from when you began

See, for one thing a diet that is not truly simple is not a good diet.

We are humans and we crave simplicity with our rituals. A diet such as the Cabbage Soup Diet that requires a specific eating regiment that *changes every day of the week* is about as inflexible and complex as can be.

Plus, did I mention you can only drink water with the rare exception of unsweetened fruit juice one day a week? Doesn't that sound like fun?

Another danger that I see, given how important I think cabbage is, is that once the Cabbage Soup Diet fails, and it will due to the excess fructose and starch and low protein it encourages, my fear is you'll never go near that healthy cabbage again!

Your Big Takeaway Tip from this Diet

My prescription for you? Eat that cabbage soup as often as you want, at any meal you want, any day you want, and try to get some fermented cabbage in the form of sauerkraut several times a week too. You'll get fantastic nutrients and good bacteria in your gut as well.

And as a bonus, the bulk in the cabbage might be good to help you feel more full... so by having a pre-entrée cabbage soup you might skip the post-entrée dessert!

Bottom line? Don't skip the cabbage or the cabbage soup... skip the Cabbage Soup Diet.

THE POCKET DIET

Probably would be better named The Portion Diet or the Pita Diet, the Pocket Diet focuses on portion sizes that you consume.

And lots and lots of pita bread.

Overview

You know what pita bread is, right? It sort of looks like the sexy croissant's half-staved, limp, empty cousin.

Pita bread opens to form a pocket that can hold other food. Pita bread pockets are not huge. The simple goal of the Pocket Diet which you are to follow for six weeks is to eat no more than will fit inside a pita bread pocket.

But before stuffing those pita bread pockets with all the potatoes and corn you can pack into them loaded with dollops of creamy sauces, there are rules in addition to the pita portion control. You have to fill your pita bread with "healthy" food such as fruits, grains, and vegetables. Fish is fine also.

Fortunately you can have non-pita snacks too but limited to some fermented foods such as yogurt as well as nuts and some cheese.

The Good...

The pita pocket keeps you from stuffing yourself. If it doesn't fit in a pita then you can't eat it. If one pita isn't enough you can't have a second.

This means that carb-heavy foods such as corn and starches that you might pack into your meals can't be such large portions that they do much damage. The Pocket Diet is certainly a calorie-counting diet with portions keeping your calories lower than they would be without the pita requirement.

The Bad and The Ugly

The designers don't seem to care about the massive amount of bread they're making you eat in the pita itself. If you can find gluten-free pita bread (I've never seen any but they make gluten-free versions of just about everything else) you at least rid yourself of the possibility of adding allergy problems to your diet.

Your Big Takeaway Tip from this Diet

Portion control is important if you want to eat virtually anything you want. Why add to your body's caloric and grain burden however by eating everything inside pita bread? Skip the pita bread and you free up a few more calories that you can make up with something else you really wanted. You won't get the heavy grain hit if you skip the pita pockets too.

In addition, the six-week limitation of the Pocket Diet means that you must change your eating plan once you finish the Pocket Diet. Any "diet" that is not truly a long-term eating plan sets you up for failure when you "end" the diet. Look for something that you can actually live with for the long term. Anything else deserves the name "fad diet."

THE JAPANESE DIET

The Japanese people are known for living a long time and not having an obesity problem as a group.

Their health and relatively slim bodies certainly warrant attention. It makes sense to try and figure out what they're doing.

Overview

Quality over quantity is the mantra of the Japanese Diet.

You are to eat foods that are in season and eat as fresh of foods as you can. This means, for example, eating asparagus during the asparagus growing season.

When you eat fresh, in-season foods you are to focus on eating less by focusing on small portions.

The Good...

You'll lose weight on the Japanese Diet for the same reason that you'll lose weight under the Pocket Diet and others like it: portion control is major to curb the amount of fat-producing carbs that enter your body.

If you've ever successfully switched from a processed-food eating routine to an extremely healthy and fresh regimen, you know that your body begins to work better on less food. The quality really can overcome the quantity.

If you can stick it out for the long haul.

Note: Speaking of the long haul, it has been shown that calorie reduction can extend your life, all other things being equal. Live longer by eating smaller portions is a major benefit of portion-reduction diets.

The Bad and The Ugly

Although the Japanese Diet focuses solely on healthy, in-season, fresh foods such as rice and potatoes can be almost as bad for your thighs as rich, sweet desserts.

Sadly, no dairy products are allowed including healthy, whole, raw milk. And meat, even organic fresh meat, is to be taken in moderation almost as a cheat. The nutrients in good meat are difficult to get from other sources without supplementation. The lack of protein-to-carb ratio, while not being a major weight-loss problem on this diet due to its small portions, may cause health problems if you exercise regularly, especially if you perform good weight-bearing exercises such as weight-lifting of any kind.

Your Big Takeaway Tip from this Diet

If you can manage portion controls *and* eat only healthy, fresh, unprocessed, in-season foods, you'll get no argument from me about the Japanese Diet's possibilities. Smaller portions, perhaps several times each day makes sense because gobbling a large meal all at once is shown to put on more poundage than spreading the same number of calories across time or meals on the same day.

THE P90X NUTRITION PLAN

How can any diet that sounds like a robot from Star Wars be all bad?

It turns out, the P90X Nutrition Plan isn't all bad! It has some interesting qualities.

Overview

If you read Dr. Clifford Sheats during his popular phase in the early-to-mid 1990s, you might recall his Lean Body Diet. The P90X Nutrition Plan seems to be extremely similar to the Lean Body Diet, especially in its core principles.

The P90X Nutrition Plan is said to give you a complete body recomposition in only 90 days. Fortunately, the P90X Nutrition Plan requires that you give up High Fructose Corn (HFCS) Syrup and most flour-based products which speeds not only weight loss but also helps keep your body from deteriorating through HFCS's possible dangerous side effects and flour's allergic reactions that often go undiagnosed.

You follow the P90X Nutrition Plan in three phases over a 90-day time period. (Actually 91 days because the phases end after 13 weeks, or 91 days exactly.) These three phases of P90X occur as follows:

- Phase 1: You can eat lean protein and low-carb veggies.

- Phase 2: You can add starchy carbs into your diet including pasta. You can also add low-glycemic fruit such as berries.

- Phase 3: While still concentrating on lean animal proteins and fresh, low-carb vegetables, even more quantities of carbohydrates are allowed to get you through the workouts.

The workouts?

Yep.

Rigorous exercise is required with the P90X Nutrition Plan.

The Good...

If you can follow the P90X Nutrition Plan, you will lose weight.

In addition, if you're currently addicted to sugars and starches, the P90X Nutrition Plan helps wean you off a big quantity of such bad things that you might be used to.

The massive amount of exercise needed certainly has the potential to get your body into shape. The question remains as to whether the extra carbohydrates are needed in Phase 2 to help you continue the exercises or if the exercises are needed to allow you to add such starchy carbs as pasta so soon. Still, a toned body and added muscles (yes, for women too) will make you look better in clothes, feel better, and have a stronger core which helps you throughout almost every aspect of your life from day to day.

The Bad and The Ugly

Adding in starchy carbs into any diet is suspect and doing so after only 4 weeks is quick to put fat-producing empty carb calories right back onto your thighs.

If you follow each Phase religiously, which by the way adds dreaded diet complexity making the P90X Nutrition Plan more difficult to stick to, the effect of those starchy carbs is mitigated by the lower portions and the unprocessed foods that are suggested. Still, this strict eating plan in each phase that allows you to add back carbs rather quickly combined with rigorous exercise required means quick failure for those who are not already highly skilled at eating specific food plans and following an exercise regimen regularly.

Your Big Takeaway Tip from this Diet

Only the most dedicated stay with the P90X Nutrition Plan for long.

You will see results early due to the complete lack of bad carbs in the first few weeks. This weight will be real weight loss and not just water loss. In addition, the exercise will work to get your muscles and toning agents working overtime.

If sticking-to-it isn't your middle name, however, you might find other diet plans easier to stick with. In addition, as I've said elsewhere in this book, any diet plan that ends after a fixed amount of time means that it's not an eating plan for life. Mentally, having a stop date for any diet might – and often does – encourage you to unconsciously develop a back-to-normal eating style once the diet ends. And normal is what might have gotten you into this mess in the first place!

THE O2 DIET

The O2 Diet promotes the ingestion of antioxidants and weight loss. Antioxidants are wonderful little fellas that help shield you against many diseases that are rampant today. They attack free radicals in your body which can cause all sorts of damage to your heart and organs.

Overview

The amount of good antioxidants in food and supplements is measured by a standard called ORAC which stands for *Oxygen Radical Absorbance Capacity*. The higher the ORAC rating the more antioxidants a food has.

The idea behind the O2 Diet is to eat foods with high ORAC ratings. Doing this not only helps shield you against health problems but foods high in ORAC often are healthy in other ways and (often) do not promote weight gain but actually do the opposite.

The Good...

I'll never argue against the fight against free radicals!

Foods highest in antioxidants are vegetables and fruits. The first four days of the O2 Diet you must consume enough fruits and vegetables to equal 50,000 ORAC points.

That's a lot of vegetables and fruits.

The Bad and The Ugly

If you've been eating healthy, meaning you haven't been OD'ing on fructose-based fruit juices and fruits high on the glycemic index such as oranges, you may very well get a sugar rush that you hate the first four days if you use fruits as a big part of the O2 Diet's introductory phase.

But I suppose for four days you can stand on your head if you had to.

After four days you can begin to bring in other foods including bread, and extremely lean meats. In addition soy products are encouraged.

That is the most obvious problem with The O2 Diet! Soy? If you feed soy to your husband, say goodbye to anything masculine about him after you put him on soy and a low fat diet. Soy might mess up women's hormones as well.

Your Big Takeaway Tip from this Diet

In spite of its adherence to high ORAC foods, the O2 Diet is little more than a low-fat, high grain, high fruit, and high vegetable diet. You and your family's bodies were designed to eat protein, especially animal protein and fats. There are some wonderful antioxidant-rich supplements on the market. The best might just be Astaxanthin. Take it daily and skip the low-fat diet that has been shown to be a colossal failure in almost every form it's been tried for the past 80 years.

THE NATURALLY THIN DIET

Oh if only all of us were thin and naturally thin without effort or thought!

Bethenny Frankel, star of the show called *Real Housewives of New York City* on TV (as opposed to all those phony housewives in New York City I suppose), says you can get thin naturally *without dieting!*

Overview

Moving away from a "diet" mentality is almost always a more successful approach at getting into shape than the mentality that you are "going on a diet for a while."

That is the approach of the Naturally Thin diet. Skip the diets and start an eating plan that you can live with forever, getting thin and staying that way.

Frankel stresses healthy qualities of food such as organic foods. But the biggest aspect of Naturally Thin is its portion control. Eat whatever you want as long as you try to stick to fresh, organic, and "healthy" (what she considers to be healthy) foods but just don't eat a lot of anything.

Tasting is better than gulping.

The Good...

By being able to have anything you want, at least a taste of anything, you will not feel "cheated" as many feel on most diets. If you have a craving and can satisfy that craving with a few tiny tastes, that craving is likely to be filled.

I have found that chewing thoroughly and savoring every bite of anything I eat enables me to eat far less but be just as satisfied. My stomach catches up to my mouth if I eat small portions and slowly.

The Bad and The Ugly

Portion control diets are nothing more than calorie-control diets. They often work but only because whatever unhealthy carbs you do eat end up being far smaller portions when they hit your stomach than you might otherwise find yourself eating.

My biggest problem with Naturally Thin is its promotion of grains and low-fat meats. It is primarily a vegan diet and no matter what Vegans tell you, you need animal proteins and fats in addition to whole-fat raw dairy and cage-free eggs.

Your Big Takeaway Tip from this Diet

I worry about your protein levels if you stick to the letter of the law on Naturally Thin. Finding a general eating plan that includes lots of strength-retaining and damage-repairing animal protein, while limiting grains, fruits, and fiberless starchy carbohydrates through portion control ensures your body gets more of what it needs while you still limit portions of the bad foods. In addition, the not-bad foods such as grass-fed beef and wild Alaskan salmon you can eat *as much as you want* so you won't even know you're on portion-control rationing if your diet is a good one. That's a plan you can stick to forever.

THE BANANA DIET

It is said that when The Banana Diet was introduced to the people of Japan a few years ago, it became such a hit that a severe banana shortage resulted.

So it must be good, right? The Japanese are supposed to be smart people.

But aren't they also supposed to be lean and healthy people also? Why would they feel the need to jump on The Banana Diet the way they did?

Overview

The Banana Diet says this:

> Eat only bananas and water for breakfast. The rest of the day eat, drink, and be merry because you can eat anything else you want.

Really?

What if the only thing I wanted the rest of the day is a bunch more bananas?

The Good

Bananas contain potassium. If you eat a lot of sodium, you need potassium to balance your electrolytes.

You've probably heard that too much sodium is bad for you but that isn't technically true. The truth is that a sodium/potassium imbalance is the problem... getting too much of one without the other.

Heart patients who must restrict their sodium levels are told to eat bananas for the very reason that doing so raises their potassium, thus putting their sodium/potassium balance into better equality. There might be better ways to get potassium without the fructose that bananas provide but if bananas do the job for some patients then great.

The Bad and The Ugly

Unless you've been instructed by your physician to eat more bananas then maybe, just maybe, you should do a double-take when you run across a diet that says to eat bananas *every day for every morning meal for the rest of your life and then you can eat anything else you want the rest of the day.*

Sure, the creators of The Banana Diet certainly never meant for you to eat bananas and drink water for breakfast and then live on Snickers bars the rest of the day. We all realize The Banana Diet is not carte blanche to *really* eat as much of anything as you want.

Plus, although containing fructose, bananas are some of the best fruits to give you a satisfied or "full" feeling. If you're going to eat a piece of fruit it's great to eat one that doesn't make you feel *more* hungry as many people quickly find themselves after eating apples or oranges.

But the carbo load you get from a banana breakfast sets you up for failure and fatigue soon after. With no protein to give you long-term energy, the effects of feeling full might soon be overrun by your body screaming for more energy in the form of calories.

Your Big Takeaway Tip from this Diet

The devil is in the details of *any* diet. With The Banana Diet you must drink room temperature water with the banana. And "anything else you want to eat" is quickly censored by the diet's designers when they warn you can have no dessert after your evening meal, you can't eat after 8pm, and you must be asleep by midnight.

All of which is good advice on any diet and by themselves those three limitations should help reduce weight – all things being equal – for any eating plan.

Oops. Two more things. No more dairy or alcohol. Processed dairy certainly has problems but if you have a local farm nearby who supplies you with delicious dairy products (especially with healthy whole, raw milk) then you've just eliminated a major source of energy and nutrients from your diet. And not having even a small, single glass of wine has drawbacks both socially and, yes, even for your health in the long-term if you'd otherwise have a little wine.

THE MAKER'S DIET

If losing weight and keeping it off was all about food and eating only, diets would be a lot easier. We just go on a diet, get to our ideal weight, then stay there forever.

The problem of dietary failure is usually balance. If you can't stick to the eating plan because you hate the food or it's ultimately not healthy for your body you won't lose weight in a healthy manner on that diet.

Many who have rampant emotional issues find themselves overeating in reaction to the way they feel emotionally. They don't always overeat because they are hungry but they find their waistlines just as big as though they were.

The best approach might just be approaching your eating plan from a 4-pronged perspective with only one of those prongs being the food.

That's what The Maker's Diet attempts to do.

Overview

To get healthy, fit, and stay that way, the creators of The Maker's Diet want you to address these four areas of your life:

- Your physical body

- Your spiritual soul

- Your emotional makeup

- Your mental well-being

Yes, it sounds sort of New Agey but the proponents of The Maker's Diet would say it's just the opposite of New Age. The Maker's Diet is based on some principles taught in the Bible.

Obviously the physical body is what one focuses on the most if using The Maker's Diet to lose weight and get fit. The foods promoted in The Maker's Diet are designed to detoxify you from the past's bad food habits and provide nutrition that will help guard against diseases in the future.

By adding only the good and eliminating the bad, the Maker's Diet attempts to make you feel better not only from being thinner but also because your cells are cleaner and more readily able to adapt and conquer future problems and attacks to your body. If you feel good physically you are far more likely to be able to address mental, emotional, and spiritual problems according to the Maker's Diet.

The Good

Looking at the whole package the way the Maker's Diet does adds to your chance at success. Focusing only on food as so many diets do means you can easily lose that focus the moment a Chocolate Volcano Ice Cream Delight dessert passes before your eyes on the way to the next table. By feeling good emotionally, mentally, and spiritually as well as physically your willpower is strong and you will have a far better sense of purpose.

The Maker's Diet wants you to stick to organic and unprocessed foods as much as possible. This reduces the amount of foreign baddies... pesticides and High Fructose Corn Syrup and other dietary evils that might otherwise evade your body's defenses.

In addition, the Maker's Diet promotes the use of herbal and other natural supplements to accent your diet. Even with organic foods, today's soil has been greatly drained of vitamins and minerals through improper over-farming and pesticides in the water systems. By adding supplements to the organic food, it is thought that you will be getting the level vitamins and minerals that the food might have originally had 100 or more years ago.

The Bad and The Ugly

Certainly the Maker's Diet's Biblical genesis, if I may use that term, will not be to the liking of some people.

In addition, the Maker's Diet warns against the use of pork such as bacon and shellfish such as shrimp and other crustaceans. The Bible's warning to Israel against those foods is the reason for the censorship of them on The Maker's Diet.

I would not avoid all pork and shellfish however; at least not for that reason. The triglycerides in bacon and the mercury levels in shellfish make those foods *in general* dangerous to eat in quantities other than a rare treat once in a while. But the foods themselves aren't posing the physical danger it's what is in them and how a lot of pork is raised.

If you can find organic, or even better locally-raised organic bacon and pork you'll be adding a nice meat to your family's healthy animal protein sources. The food chain called *Chipotle* guarantees that all pork they serve is made from pigs that got to roam all the grass and mud their little hearts desired and were never hormone-injected or fed a diet solely of corn. Chipotle is having such success that hopefully other places will get a hint and begin serving healthy meats such as grass-fed, hormone-free products to make it even easier to overcome the traditional problem with modern pork and other meats.

Your Big Takeaway Tip from this Diet

As you can see and as one would expect, the Maker's Diet focuses far more heavily on the physical aspect of the diet than the promised mental, emotional, and spiritual aspects. Still, the detoxification foods, the suggested supplements, and the overall approach of becoming more aware of potential problems that may be active in your body and soul, is not a bad recipe for a healthy lifestyle.

THE KETOGENIC DIET

The Ketogenic Diet appears to have benefits besides weight loss. The Ketogenic Diet is said to be a helpful eating regimen for those who suffer from epilepsy, a neurological disorder that brings with it seizures and other possible brain problems.

Way back in the 1920s a Ketogenic Diet was designed and proved helpful to epilepsy sufferers but the drug companies decided they had a better way. "Eat what you want as long as you pop our pill to control your seizures." (In fairness they are not that direct, but I am highly suspicious of any med that replaces results from a good diet.)

The Ketogenic Diet has once again gained favor in recent years as the turn away from a dependence on drugs once again looks at possible dietary approaches to our health problems.

Overview

The Ketogenic Diet is a low-carb diet without a doubt. The word *ketogenic* almost always implies a low-carb, high-fat, high protein diet and applies in some way to a few of the more popular diets and books you may have heard of in the past 2 decades such as Atkins, The 4-Hour Body, and to a big extent the South Beach Diet.

When you eat only a few carbohydrates, your body has to begin using fat stored on your thighs and hips and waist for energy. And that means we have less fat! On a high-carb diet your body will utilize any carbs in your body and ignore your fat stores that it thinks, "I'll just keep those fat cells in a safe and secure place all over those thighs in case I find myself stuck in the middle of the Arctic without food for a few weeks!"

So on a low-carb diet your body makes far better use of what it has for energy and you lose fat and weight. Hardly any ketogenic-based diet is complete without a good source of animal protein and fats.

The Ketogenic Diet also wants exercise to play a role in your lifestyle while you maintain the Ketogenic Diet. As many as 5 days of aerobics are required.

The Good...

You need good, healthy animal protein to lose weight easily, retain a good form, reduce accidents in your bones and muscles, build strong bodies for exercise, and to fight diseases as they begin to attack you.

It's no secret to the actual researchers of diets that a "good lubing" is essential so get good fats such as healthy animal fats, essential fatty acids such as ground flaxseed (men don't always do well with flaxseed oil by the way unless it's said to have a high count of "lignans" which some brands such as Barleans contains), fish oil, and the oils you get from cold water fish.

Healthy fats not only come from the oils but also good sources are nuts and vegetables such as avocadoes.

Note: Just to be clear, eating fat does *not* make you fat! You can disagree with me and agree with the government's food recommendations all you want. Just keep in mind the government is comprised of the same people who brought you the Driver of Motor Vehicles (DMV) and the TSA at the airports. Research promptly shows that the government's food advice got a tremendous make-over that hurt all of us when George McGovern, after losing the Presidential election by the largest margin ever, was put in charge of the "McGovern Report" written by a committee of professing animal rights activists. I would say that their scientific research had flaws but that would be falsely implying that any science was actually present in any manner on that committee.

The Ketogenic Diet promotes all this kind of food and steers you toward a ketogenic state where your body is highly efficient at burning off the fat.

The Bad and The Ugly

No starchy carbs are allowed *except* you can load more carbohydrates into your system on weekends. When you overeat after being on a low-carbohydrate diet your body counteracts what can become a leptin deficiency which can affect women's menstruation.

That is why your weekends really should reverse course with a bit of fruit, maybe some gluten-free-based pizza, and even an organic potato if you really must. The Ketogenic Diet says you can add in these extra carbs on the weekends but as Tim Ferriss found out you have a much higher chance at success if you limit this to just one day a week. Plus your leptin levels will remain fine at this level of eating.

This means no desserts for most of your week. No sugar of any kind. No fruit juice and virtually no fruit unless you stick with low-carb, high glycemic fruits such as berries.

Aerobics are beginning to come under scrutiny as not being as good as it has been touted the past 40 years since Dr. Kenneth Cooper, M.D. developed the concept. Not only are joint problems occurring in many but the heart and lymphatic systems just might not be designed to take high intensity aerobic exercise for more than a few minutes at a time.

Your Big Takeaway Tip from this Diet

I like the Ketogenic Diet. I'd modify it from two days of high carbs down to just one. One is enough to keep your leptin in check. In addition, I warn you strongly against 5 days of aerobic exercises each week. Not only do *most* find that level of activity unsustainable (thereby quitting all exercise) but new research is screaming at us describing the benefits of interval aerobics.

Look into some of what Dr. Al Sears, M.D., has developed with the PACE program. This basically involves exercising for as little as *10 minutes* to get the same results as 30-to-45 minutes of high-intensity aerobics. His PACE program and others like it suggest you do low-heart rate exercise such as walking for 2-3 minutes followed by high-intensity power-walking or even running if your body can take it for a minute or so. Then alternate this 3-minute walking with 1-minute high-heart rate aerobic exercise for 4 or 5 times. The result is a far greater fat loss than seen otherwise.

Dr. John Ratey, M.D. describes near the end of his book *Spark* that this kind of interval exercise was the only way he could lose the last few pounds of fat from around his trouble area: the belly.

THE HUNGRY GIRL DIET

Hey girls, surely you remember that Cyndi Lauper song called, *Girls Just Want to Have Lunch!* (Okay, maybe it was Weird Al Yankovich...?)

Anyway it's true isn't it? We love to get together with our gal pals and have lunch and talk and talk and have lunch!

Sounds to me like a diet named the Hungry Girl Diet was designed just for us.

Overview

What food do you like to eat most?

If your answer is Triple Ripple Fudge Cake with Quadruple Maple Toffee Topping, maybe I should have you back up and *really* think about it. What food do you like to eat most?

Well, even if you insist it *is* that kind of dessert, the Hungry Girl Diet is going to let you eat it. Isn't that great?

The only difference is that you'll have to prepare your yummy dessert in a much different way from what you're used to. And let me assure you that it won't *quite* taste the same. But you can still have your cake and eat it too!

The Hungry Girl Diet says eat whatever food you like to eat. Just make it in a manner that causes the least amount of damage to your system. The Hungry Girl Diet is more about *how* you prepare your food and less about *what* food you eat.

The Good...

Admit it, any diet that lets us eat what we like is something we're interested in.

The Hungry Girl Diet's creator, author Lisa Lillien, provides step-by-step recipes that train you how to reduce calories in food you already eat so the food's impact is far less on your thighs and hubby's waist.

Being a Nutritionist, Lillien strives to replace the bad with good stuff, maintaining anything she considers healthy in the original food you like and if possible replacing the bad with less bad or far better ingredients.

The Bad and The Ugly

Lillien suggests sugar substitutes and unless you use Stevia, you might want to wean yourself off the sweeteners. Although *local*, organic honey does offer you some health benefits don't overdo it if you decide to use honey. And if you opt for store-bought honey you're not doing your body any favor… as with "Grade A" Maple Syrup, is full of garbage that harm you more than they taste good.

Note: Organic locally-farmed honey has some good immunity-boosting and antibacterial properties so a spoonful every few days is a tasty maintenance pick-me-up. But honey is pure sugar and other than a little taste now and then "for medicinal purposes only" of course, keep your paws off the local, organic honey. If you and your family must cheat and have some maple syrup on carb-laden pancakes and waffles once in a blue moon, why not get the *good* and *real* stuff and skip the dangerous garbage sold as "syrup" today? You can find organic Grade B maple syrup if you look closely at many of today's grocery stores, especially the better ones such as Whole Foods. The benefits of this *real* maple syrup outweigh the sugar properties as long as you really do reserve it for very special and few-and-far between days.

Many of Lillien's food preparation recipes attempt to take the fat out of many dishes. This can actually work against you more than leaving the fat in. Fat in food can lower the glycemic qualities of the food making them harder to stay on your thighs. For example, putting real, organic, homemade butter from whole, raw milk cream on a slice of warm, organic, fresh-ground wheat bread results in that piece of bread doing far less damage than it would without the butter.

Your Big Takeaway Tip from this Diet

There's nothing wrong with looking at Hungry Girl Diet recipes to get some good food preparation tips. You will find ways to avoid calories that otherwise might enter your stomach. Be cautious that you don't overdo artificial sweeteners (better yet, avoid them altogether or use Stevia) and lowering animal or real dairy fat too much can work against your weight as much as it can work for you.

THE NO S DIET

At first glance, the No S Diet might make you think it stands for something it doesn't.

But have no fear, you can discuss the No S Diet with your own grandmother because it is easy to follow as long as you keep three little S's out of your eating routine.

Overview

The S's in the No S Diet are:

- Sugar

- Snacks

- Seconds

As you've seen in this book alone, dieticians disagree about as much as the countries in the Middle East but there is hardly one of them who would offer much argument against the three S's of the No S Diet.

But wait there's more! On weekends (the only days of the week that begin with the letter S by the way!) you can eat the three S's again. Also, Special occasions such as holidays are also okay to have one or more of the S's.

The Good...

The No S Diet is a combination of portion control and carb control.

The portions are controlled through the no seconds. The carbs are controlled through the disappearance of sugar and snacks. And don't cheat, you *know* by now that most fruit and starchy veggies are thinly-veiled versions of sugar because those simple carbs break down into sugars quickly once you've eaten them. The same is true of milk but raw, whole milk contains enzymes that the homogenization and pasteurization processes haven't destroyed making that milk's casein a less threatening sugar if you don't overdo it. But if you get regular store-bought milk, then it's off limits so remember that.

The No S Diet also promotes healthy animal protein such as fish, chicken, and beef. Also eggs and cheese are fine along with other proteins such as cottage cheese.

The Bad and The Ugly

It's rare to find a diet that promotes animal proteins *and* breads, grains, and therefore cereals but the No S Diet does. The only problem with diets that are portion control diets is you never want to limit portions of good, healthy protein that comes from organic and grass-fed sources and cold water fish low in mercury.

Also, the No S Diet promotes "lean" meats which deprive you of many healthy fats that will not only lube your innards as Granny used to say but also are needed for a healthy balance.

Keep an eye on your complex carbohydrates such as pastas and starchy vegetables such as corn and potatoes. If you follow the No S Diet strictly those are legal foods but if you can, try not to make those complex carbs a daily part of your diet. They tend to turn to sugar fairly rapidly in your body which somewhat violates the No Sugar plank of the No S Diet.

Your Big Takeaway Tip from this Diet

Overall, the No S Diet gets a grade of A from me. As you may have gleaned from this book, I think research tends to favor a low-carb diet as one that is easiest to stick to and lose weight on but I think the No S Diet will work for many people who have failed at lots of other diet attempts in the past.

THE FAT LOSS 4 LIFE DIET

So, who is going to admit they need a diet called the *Fat Loss 4 Idiots Diet*?

Actually, the Fat Loss 4 Idiots Diet is one that requires that its followers be fairly strict and disciplined. Also, using "intuition" when making food choices is suggested.

One would think that an idiot's intuition is not to be trusted! So, can the Fat Loss 4 Idiots Diet be trusted? Let's find out.

Overview

The Fat Loss 4 Idiots Diet only lasts two weeks.

During that time you are to eat a wide variety of specific foods in an effort to stir your metabolism and ramp it up to high gear for weight burning. The stated goals of the Fat Loss 4 Idiots Diet are almost one full pound a day.

The intuition part of the Fat Loss 4 Idiots Diet is in portion control. You are to use common sense, incorrectly called "intuition," when doling out portions of your meals.

The Good...

After 11 days of sticking to the specific eating plan of four small meals each day spaced not too far apart, you get three binge days where you can eat whatever you want. To be fair, they aren't binge days when it comes to quantity because you are to eat whatever you want until you get close to full.

The dietary plan is similar to the old Lean Bodies diet where you eat lean animal proteins, eggs, and non-starchy vegetables.

The Bad and The Ugly

Besides the adherence to "lean" meats which can raise concern about how many healthy fats you are keeping out of your diet, the Fat Loss 4 Idiots Diet also incorporates fruits and grains such as whole cereals and oatmeal into its regimen. In reality this means you're eating a low-fat diet not dissimilar to many others. And low-fat diets don't do too well in the "and I kept it off forever" category.

Your Big Takeaway Tip from this Diet

Don't be an idiot! Avoid the Fat Loss 4 Idiots Diet!

Actually, there are far worse diets out there, many are described in this book. But in general a low-fat diet, especially one that is scheduled to end after so many days, will probably give you short-term weight loss at the expense of not enjoying yourself during the process and returning to your previous ways of weight gain afterwards.

THE EAT TO LIVE DIET

The Eat to Live Diet sounds good!

Let's eat to live and not live to eat. As pleasurable as food is, and as pleasurable as food *should be*, other things in life should define us. Our waist size should not be the measurement of how successful we are at our hopes and dreams.

Overview

The Eat to Live Diet basically boils down to eating as healthy of food as possible. What is healthy to one may not be healthy to someone else as we'll see.

Still, with any eating plan, you always stack benefits on top of another if you eat the best quality of food you can while following the eating plan you have determined is the best for you. Along those same lines, the Eat to Live Diet says you should strive for nutrient-rich foods and you are given two choices:

1. The vegetarian plan

2. The limited animal protein plan.

The Good...

Many of us agree that it's not just about the food we eat but it's the source of the food we eat. If you stick with organic foods you reduce the existence of pesticides in your body. If you stick with locally-grown food sources as much as possible, some rather interesting studies have shown that eating "close to home" has added health benefits.

So whatever eating plan or diet you decide, the Eat to Live Diet is 100% correct. If you're going to eat veggies, make them organic! If you're going to eat meat, make it grass-fed beef and cold-water fish that is less prone to have mercury traces in it.

Cooking almost always destroys *some* nutrients too. So don't overcook your veggies and don't char your meat. (Even though charred meat can sure be good!) The Eat to Live Diet promotes a fresh and uncooked diet when possible.

Note: With rare exception you should heat all your foods less. Sauerkraut for example contains far more probiotics if you make it yourself using the extremely simple cold press method as opposed to most that you buy in jars and (ugh!) BPA-plastic-lined cans that has been heated. Tomatoes actually increase in nutrients after being cooked! Isn't that interesting? But in general the fresher and the less heated the better.

The Bad and The Ugly

The promoters of the Eat to Live Diet sure like to promote the vegetarian plan over the limited animal protein plan. And like so many others like it, eating lean meats and very little of them reduces healthy and needed oils and fats in your system.

In addition, the Eat to Live Diet stresses breads and grains and a long list of other items that add carb poundage to your thighs and hips.

Your Big Takeaway Tip from this Diet

Whenever you eat, whatever you choose, wherever you go, always increase the benefit of your food by eating as healthy of ingredients as possible. Opt for raw vegetables over cooked. Opt for medium or even rare beef over well done. If you must eat bread, do the work and grind organic wheat into flour right before you bake your own bread. That kind of bread has lots of benefits in spite of the carbs but be sure and butter it liberally with homemade, organic butter to slowdown the glycemic impact.

Other than the healthy ingredients, the Eat to Live Diet doesn't offer a lot of long-term success promise. It's like so many other low-fat, heavy vegetarian diets.

THE DIET SOLUTION PROGRAM

What type are you? You have to find out if you want to follow the Diet Solution Program.

Overview

The Diet Solution Program classifies everybody into these three types:

1. Protein

2. Carbohydrates

3. Protein and carbohydrates

Once you learn what your dietary type is, the Diet Solution Program provides one of three diets for you. Obviously these diets are heavy in protein or heavy in carbohydrates or both.

The Good...

Not everybody eats the same way. Not everybody reacts to food the same way. And not everybody loses weight the same way.

Fortunately, patterns develop that work overall such as starchy carbs being bad, sugar being bad, and so on. But the Diet Solution Program attempts to find out more about the type of eater you are and formulates a diet to best suit you. This has a lot of appeal because you're more likely to lose weight if your type has truly and accurately been established. (This assumes the three types defined by the Diet Solution Program are actually real scientifically provable types that people fall into.)

By adhering to the diet type plan you're given for your type, you should lose weight and maybe stick with that eating plan for life. The Diet Solution Program promotes nutrient rich foods and fresh and uncooked vegetables which is always a plus. In addition, the Diet Solution Program is one of the few (surprisingly) that warns you away from processed soy and bad fats (such as hydrogenated fats) which I'm always a fan of you avoiding.

The Bad and The Ugly

If you are a vegan now, don't get typed! You might find out that the lifestyle you chose doesn't match the diet you should be eating. And can I be frank? I concur with that without even knowing your type.

Your Big Takeaway Tip from this Diet

I don't know the percentages of people who fall in the different types but it's my suspicion most people are typed as protein and a protein/carb mix type. While promoting healthy organic and unprocessed ingredients as much as possible while warning against soy, the Diet Solution Program has little I can find that is a problem.

THE hGC DIET

Somehow this diet has been around since the 1950s and still gets press and some followers. I'll spend a little more time on it than most of the other crash diets here due to its two-pronged gotcha - if you like to starve yourself and get lots of injections you'll *love* the hGC Diet!

Overview

The hGC Diet gets its name from the hormone called human *chrorionic gonadotrophin*. This is a hormone pregnant women produce naturally.

To adhere to the hGC Diet's premise you must:

1. Dramatically restrict your calorie intake to fewer than 500 calories a day.

2. Get daily injections of hGC.

Some offshoots of the hGC Diet have been proposed such as a more homeopathic approach but these seem to change the diet enough so that it isn't truly the hGC Diet any longer as it was designed. Plus, the results in general have been even less than stellar than those who following the actual hGC Diet getting the shots.

The Good...

You lose some weight. You also lose weight if you saw your legs off your body.

The Bad and The Ugly

You get a double whammy with the hGC diet!

Both calorie restriction and the hGC hormone injections are hotly debated among the medical and dietary establishments.

Calorie restriction, especially when the calories that you restrict are starchy carbs, will certainly drop the pounds from you. Whether you take the hormone injections or not, nobody debates whether the calorie restriction part of the hGC Diet works.

The debate comes in when one begins to discuss the long-term weight loss as well as the health problems with severe calorie restriction.

You've heard time and time again that most who go on a crash diet, which usually means limited calories, do lose weight only to gain all the weight back and more as soon as they go off the diet. You don't need a study to prove this though do you? Both you and I have calorie restricted diets at some time in our lives, sometimes multiple times, and we know the results after we stop... and *we always stop*!

The reason we stop is that it's so unnatural to limit our calories in a severe manner. It also is counter-productive in spite of the fact that we do lose initial weight.

Why?

Gary Taubes in his excellent book *Why We Get Fat* looks at the behavioral aspects of severe calorie restriction diets. He asks what you would do if you were given a free dinner of your choice at the best place on earth? You will be getting all you can eat of your ultimate favorite appetizers, entrées, side dishes, breads, and desserts. Yum!

How would you prepare for the biggest and best feast of your life?

You'd certainly not eat much during the day! And you might limit what you eat a few days before too. In other words, you naturally prepare to overeat by not eating beforehand! You willfully restrict your calories so your body can jump into that meal that is going to be so tasty and massive.

This is what you do when you restrict your calories. Not only do you risk not getting enough nutrients your body yearns for but you also are setting yourself up for a bloat-fest when you can't stand the lack of calories any longer.

We've all done this to some extent. I, personally, am sad to say I was on a calorie-depravation diet as a teenaged girl and I lasted for two and a half months during summer and I got to be thin as a rail by the time school started... and I was miserable both in how I felt, how I acted, and yes, how I looked!

I began eating the first day of school like I hadn't eaten in... well, in two and a half months! And I was pudgy by early November once again.

Hormone injections. Daily?

Do we *really* need to say much here?

If you've seen any women's health news over the past decade you know that hormones have proved to be tricky at best in solving women's problems and often cause severe troubles.

Calorie restriction, especially when the calories that you restrict are starchy carbs, will certainly drop the pounds from you. Whether you take the hormone injections or not, nobody debates whether the calorie restriction part of the hGC Diet works. The danger can lie also in the hormone shots. You know this.

Just take the basics: Do you want your arms or hips to look (and feel) like a junkie's before the month is over? Daily injections... Yes, as often as daily for your hGC injections.

That sounds like a lot of fun and money, right?

Plus, the hGC is a restricted substance so you need a prescription. hGC is often used as an infertility hormone and certainly there are good reasons to correct the hormone imbalance with women who have fertility issues. But does being overweight mean you have a hormone imbalance? Or a sugar-in-the-mouth imbalance?

Does it work? The goal of the hGC injection is to curb your appetite. When you limit yourself to a potentially dangerous 500 calories a day, you'd better do something to curb your appetite or risk going crazy. (I would go crazy on 500 calories a day!)

Your Big Takeaway Tip from this Diet

Keep in mind the hGC Diet was introduced in the 1950s so we have decades of studies about it.

And according to Dr. Oz, a man with whom I don't always agree with, it's difficult to argue that over a dozen trials have been made, all centered around the hGC Diet, often replacing the hGC with a salt-fluid injected placebo, and the resulting weight loss numbers were *no better* than using the expensive, side-effect potential, costly hGC hormone injection.

THE COCONUT DIET

A few years ago, a politically-driven food group ostentatiously calling themselves the Center for Science in the Public Interest (CSPI) called for the ban of coconut oil on movie theater popcorn. As usual, the CSPI got it wrong; it is the starchy popcorn grain that is the real danger in that combination.

But it does taste good, especially when popped in coconut oil!

It is said that the *last man standing* is the winner. Coconuts and coconut oil are not only still standing but making a comeback like never before! The health benefits of coconut oil are making the headlines these days and the Coconut Diet is jumping on the health bandwagon too.

Overview

The Coconut Diet works to accentuate the benefits of coconuts and their oils. This tropical fruit is praised by both carbohydrate supporters as well as low-carb crowd as an excellent health benefactor and a wonderful way to cook many of the foods you never considered cooking in coconut oil.

Am I a fan? Just this morning I cooked myself two organic cage-free eggs over-easy in a cast iron skillet of coconut oil. Yumm!

Note: Do you have easy-to-use, non-stick Teflon pans? When does your garbage get picked up because those need to be tossed immediately! The health maladies related to that kind of "easy" cookware is being revealed more and more. Why take a chance? Your grandmother and great-grandmother used cast iron skillets for everything and millions of grandmas can't be wrong!

The Coconut Diet is more than just cooking foods in the oil however. It requires four stages:

1. The Kickoff which lasts for three weeks and consists of animal proteins and non-starchy vegetables. Nope, no fruit or sugars but that's almost always fine.

2. Cleansing where you boost your fiber considerably. And for those of you who love a thrill, the creators of the Coconut Diet suggest that you undergo a colonic!

3. Carbs are now added back into your diet including grains and some fruits. I'd avoid making this a huge change over what you've been doing so far.

4. Maintenance that you can continue to remain on as long as you wish but still no sugar and limited fruit intake.

All along the way you will be taking three tablespoons of coconut oil, perhaps in a drink or as a dressing. I'd not hesitate to suggest you cook as much with it too.

The Good...

The Coconut Diet is good about requiring that the coconut oil you use is as healthy as possible. You'll want to find organic coconut oil and extra virgin is best in my opinion.

Coconut oil is one of the most rapid energy creators you can ingest. Instead of moving directly to our thighs it is ready-to-use as an instant energy source. In addition among its health benefits are immunity boosting elements.

Although lean meats are encouraged, the coconut oil does help alleviate the problems of not getting enough animal fats in your diet by providing you with the energy-boosting coconut oil. I'd still suggest not worrying too much about sticking with lean meats only since fat doesn't make you fat. As always, grass-fed organic beef and cold water fish and cage-free chicken makes your animal fats far more healthy than they are straight from a typical supermarket's shelf.

The Bad and The Ugly

Daily exercise is required although not a large amount. So know in advance this is not just a diet but also a diet and exercise program.

Also, the Coconut Diet isn't the easiest one to follow. Simplicity is always preferred when possible and the Coconut Diet has some rather specific requirements that you might find difficult to follow depending on your work or travel schedule.

I'll leave it as an exercise to the reader to decide if the colonic in the second phase is to be considered a Good or a Bad.

Your Big Takeaway Tip from this Diet

I really like the foundations of the Coconut Diet and I rarely like any diet that focuses heavily on one specific food. Having said that, I promote the theory that a diet that is simple to follow is one that *will* be followed. The Coconut Diet isn't simple. If you decide not to adopt the Coconut Diet, I'd still suggest you find some of that delicious, organic, extra-virgin coconut oil and use it in as much food preparation as you are able.

THE FRUITARIAN DIET

Want to save the environment at the expense of you and your family's health?

Then join the revolution and adopt the Fruitarian Diet.

Overview

Sugar, sugar everywhere - not a muscle remains to employ it... Perhaps you've noticed from my poem... I'm not a fan of this diet!

The Fruitarian Diet says skip the healthy, needed animal protein and fat and forgo the incredibly delicious products available at your local organic dairy. Instead you will eat nuts, seeds, and fruits with seeds so the plant "doesn't have to die" as would be the case with say a carrot (I am not making this up).

If you're feeling extremely nasty, a vegetable with seeds can be tossed into your stomach as long as you don't cook it or eat it with any other fruit or vegetable at the same time.

To (try) to live by the Fruitarian Diet you are required to ensure that no animal or plant has to die so that you can live.

Again... I am not making this up.

The Good...

Fruit tastes good, that's for sure.

Nuts and seeds have some good oils and fats that your body needs.

And an almost 100% pure sugar diet will really get your engine going. Until you crash at which time you eat more sugar in the next piece of seed-based fruit you choose.

Plus you save on electricity and gas since you're not allowed to cook anything.

The Bad and The Ugly

No animal protein means your children's muscles have a huge chance to develop too slowly, giving your adolescent boys the upper body strength of their toddler sisters.

Sickness and disease have a good chance to take over your family's bodies since there is no protein to stand guard and help repair tissue damage.

You will be spending a lot of money on dietary supplements to replace the vitamins and minerals your body *requires* that you don't get on the Fruitarian Diet.

Note: Seriously, is there anything about this thing I like? It has been shown that if you come down with an illness such as the flu that a simple fruit and fruit juice diet, taken in small doses but basically fasting even from much of that, can allow your body to kick in some natural defenses and get you well without the need of meds. But the fruit isn't doing the action, it's the energy otherwise going to digesting food that allows your body to repair. Still, if you don't have the foundational vitamins and minerals that a *balanced diet provides* then there isn't much for your body to work with during such a fruit-based fast.

Your Big Takeaway Tip from this Diet

The biggest benefit to the environment you might make if you adopt a pure Fruitarian Diet is the large number of bacterial elements in the soil that your early-to-grave body provides the bugs and crawly things as your coffin disintegrates six feet under.

Ok, I'm being overly dramatic. But still… don't do this diet!

THE HAY DIET

No it's *not* a diet where you eat a bunch of hay!

It's called that because its founder's name was William H. Hay and he created the Hay Diet 100 years ago.

Overview

The entire premise behind Dr. Hay's diet is that certain foods are never to be eaten together or you'll have all sorts of trouble. His foundation for the Hay Diet was the pH factor of food. pH determines how acidic or alkaline a substance is. Dr. Hay's theory was that you could eat alkaline foods or acidic foods but never eat them at the same time in the same meal.

Note: Some foods are considered neutral and can be eaten with either of the other types.

The Good...

Dr. Hay was suffering from at least one illness and got better by sticking with this theory of dieting. A side effect was that he lost weight.

If pH does play a role in digestion then your body probably absorbs food nutrients better if you stick to one end of the pH scale or the other. Also perhaps you will digest such a single type of food better.

The Bad and The Ugly

Some of the Hay Diet is confusing. For example, while animal proteins are considered acidic so are flour-based breads, grains, and sugar. Yet, you can't combine bread and meat in the same meal. This complexity not only causes the diet to begin to be confusing but it also seems to violate the very premise of the diet.

In addition, a vegetarian meal is to be preferred more often over that an acidic meat-based diet so Dr. Hay would have you eating greens more than meats for your daily meals.

Your Big Takeaway Tip from this Diet

Did Dr. Hay get better because of his diet or did he get better *while* trying his diet? Clinical studies have not shown the Hay Diet to be extremely reliable.

THE ORNISH DIET

Dr. Dean Ornish created his Ornish Diet several years ago.

The diet is a low-fat eating regimen.

Overview

Tons of food are off limits when you give the Ornish Diet a try. The reason is that the Ornish Diet attempts to eliminate fat from your diet. Also, sugar is forbidden in spite of its low-fat nature.

This eliminates not only meats and many vegetables such as avocados but also nuts.

Dr. Ornish doesn't like you touching low-fat or non-fat versions of dairy or cheese either. What a Grinch!

The Good...

The lack of sugar certainly is a plus for any diet. Also, Dr. Ornish says that it's better to eat multiple meals with smaller portions than fewer large-portion meals each day.

The Bad and The Ugly

One plank of the Ornish Diet is that you must be in the gym 30 minutes a day exercising. Your poor muscles are going to get a pounding without the lubricating effects of fat and without the protein of a non-meat diet.

Dr. Ornish ignores the massive research for animal fats or healthy essential oils and nuts and insists that his research shows that a non-fat diet will make you healthier and leaner.

Your Big Takeaway Tip from this Diet

Gary Taubes in his *Why We Get Fat* shows study after study and clinical trial results right and left showing the weight-loss and major health benefits of animal proteins and good fats and oils. It appears that Dr. Ornish disagrees with the doctors that Taubes cites considerably. If you're a vegetarian you probably will do better under the Ornish Diet than the Fruitarian Diet.

THE FRENCH WOMEN DON'T GET FAT DIET

Yes they do, I've been to France!

The French Women Don't Get Fat Diet has one of the best names of all the diets out there. I love it!

But should we follow the dietary patterns of French women? Should we ladies also stop shaving our armpits the way they do over there too?

Overview

How do the French do it? They eat heavy, creamy, rich sauces on their foods. They eat lots of cheese. They love French bread.

The French, as with the Italians, take their food seriously. And they do this by insisting on high quality and fresh contents in their meals. Sadly, our processed and fast food culture had begun to appear in Europe and has started to show its effects on their health.

Overall, however, they do seem to have less of a weight problem than we do; they are over there eating all that "good stuff" that seems to go right to our thighs.

The Good...

The French Women Don't Get Fat Diet requires that you limit yourself to small portions and chew slowly. That way you not only get the great taste that fresh and organic and unprocessed foods can provide but you also feel full faster because your stomach has a chance to catch up to your mouth and send a "I'm done" signal before you've downed that third *Royale with Cheese* or a *Le Big Mac*.

Yogurt is highly recommended since French women supposedly eat a lot of yogurt. Homemade yogurt made from fresh, raw, whole milk is one of the best things you can do for your stomach. As I like to say, "Fix your gut and fix your health."

You can even enjoy some wine and dessert but you must severely limit your portions.

The Bad and The Ugly

The French Women Don't Get Fat Diet requires portion control like no other. The high carbohydrate combination with all the proteins and fats is a recipe for disaster if you don't want the portions. That means it's actually a calorie-counting diet without the actual counting.

Your Big Takeaway Tip from this Diet

If you fail at diets that are extra strict and if you like REAL yogurt (I don't like it but I eat it daily; you should too!), you might do very well the rest of your life living like the Mademoiselles live so give the French Women Don't Get Fat Diet a try.

THE EAT CLEAN DIET

As you may have guessed from its name, the Eat Clean Diet is a diet based on eating foods that are high quality but also you are to eat them in their unprocessed, natural form.

Overview

On the Eat Clean Diet, raw is better than cooked. Cooked lightly is better than cooked heavily.

If it comes in a box with lots of added ingredients, it isn't allowed on the Eat Clean Diet.

The Good...

The Eat Clean Diet has a lot of truth and science behind it. Certainly cooking can destroy the nutrients in many foods. In addition, processed foods have hardly *any* of their original nutrient content unless the food company adds back a bunch of synthetic vitamins and minerals replacing the natural ones they took out processing your food. (Think white Wonder Bread. Think pasteurized, homogenized milk. Yuck and yuck!)

The Eat Clean Diet promotes the idea that multiple small meals throughout your day is better than a few large ones.

The Bad and The Ugly

You may not see extremely rapid results but all in all that is okay and often preferably to rapid weight loss.

Your Big Takeaway Tip from this Diet

If portion control has been a problem before, you may really like the Eat Clean Diet. You can basically eat as much of the legal foods as you wish and probably still lose weight. You should follow the yogurt suggestion to get your probiotics although staying away from processed foods is a great step towards keeping your stomach's good bacteria.

The Eat Clean Diet stresses a little too much leanness for my taste – lean meat, egg whites only, etc., which has been show to slow down instead of ramping up weight loss (eat whole eggs, not egg whites!!) but in general if you can maintain a natural food lifestyle you will enjoy the Eat Clean Diet.

THE BABY FOOD DIET

Lose the baby fat and eat the baby food...

If you have no teeth, this might be right up your alley!

Overview

Eat nothing but baby food.

You heard that right.

You know, the stuff in the little jars that you *act as though* it's good when you force it into your little one's mouth.

Hmmm... let's chew on this a while longer.

The Good

Baby foods typically have fewer processed substances than other foods. In addition, Baby foods are pureed and easy to digest. That means there is no solid, or no solids large enough to require chewing.

Babies whose teeth haven't developed obviously need this kind of food.

And if you are feeding your baby *organic* baby food, and even better making your own baby food from grass-fed and organic sources, then you're little child is getting exactly what he or she is going to need to develop strong teeth.

If *you're* going to try The Baby Food Diet you certainly should use only organic baby food also. Again, making your own is the best way to ensure you're eating truly healthy food.

The Bad and The Ugly

But you already have teeth. At least that's going to be my assumption here.

And there's a good reason why you have teeth... it's so you can bite into those delicious fresh vegetables and grass-fed beef and low-glycemic berries and chew on those wonderful organic nuts.

You *can* puree all your food before eating it. But then you could just pour it into a glass and drink it.

But you will quickly find that *chewing* is one of the reasons we are satisfied when we eat! The process of chewing not only prepares the food for our stomachs to break down further but the chewing of food actually increases our saliva flow and our stomach acid. This *prepares* our stomachs better for food so our stomach linings can absorb the nutrients and eliminate waste.

Chewing also makes food taste good. The actual taste of a bite of sizzling grass-fed steak changes as you chew through the layers of beef. The tastes of healthy, wholesome, non-starchy organic vegetables change as you bite into them, producing an array of tastes you will never get if you eat baby food or pre-pureed all your food to begin with.

In other words, you'll hate eating the stuff after too long.

Your Big Takeaway Tip from this Diet

Keep in mind, a big advantage of baby food is that it is said not to be processed as much as other foods can be. (You'd better make sure of these claims for your baby's sake by the way. Making your own is always best.) In addition, baby food doesn't have as much sugar or additives as the processed foods we can buy. You can even get gluten-free baby food if you have a problem with allergies or think you might have a problem with allergies.

But every one of those benefits is true of any and all healthy food that you should be eating.

By limiting yourself to baby food, you are paying far more for the same food you'd get elsewhere in larger quantities. The only advantage is it comes in little jars you can use later for make-up I suppose!

Real food – it's what your teeth were designed for.

THE CHOCOLATE DIET

Get out of my way and show me where I sign up for the Chocolate Diet!!!

You ladies know what I mean, right? Sometimes nothing works as well as chocolate. And we've always been told how bad that evil, poisonous, sinful, scrumptious, delicious chocolate is for us.

But perhaps... is there a chance that chocolate has been given a bad rap?

Overview

The Chocolate Diet lasts for two weeks. On it, you're promised to lose weight while not giving up that delightful brown magical substance – Proof that miracles can happen.

On the Chocolate Diet you are allowed to eat chocolate because the thought is that if told to give it up completely, you'd go nuts *and* quit the diet anyway. All the Chocolate Diet asks is that you stop chocolate for seven days. Seven... long... days. And then, perhaps your cravings will be diminished somewhat so that a much smaller portion than our typical pound-of-brown cravings require.

The Good...

You are to take supplements to help ease the cravings of food and chocolate. I'm all for supplements as long as you get natural supplements from reliable sources. A high quality liquid vitamin and mineral supplement that you take an ounce or so daily is always a nice way to get lots with less effort. You'll still need to supplement with some capsules such as vitamin D3 and calcium. Ask a homeopath doctor what they recommend. Or ask your M.D. and do the opposite. Ha!

The Bad and The Ugly

The Chocolate Diet requires that you watch calories and abide by a low-cal diet. This means lots of veggies and skim milk. The lack of fat in the milk may make your cravings for some comfort food (meaning, yes, chocolate!) stronger however.

Your Big Takeaway Tip from this Diet

If you're truly having a chocolate problem, the Chocolate Diet can turn you from a raging chocoholic into a slightly slender, less raging chocoholic. The chance that this diet will cure us of this wondrous devilish delight is slimmer than you and my waists cut down halfway. It is said that dark chocolate provides some health benefits in the form of some fermentation-like properties. (Too bad because I prefer the milk chocolate.) So if you must cheat, see if the dark chocolate can satisfy you.

Once your cravings are reduced from the Chocolate Diet consider going on a lifelong eating plan that does not count calories or remove a lot of fats from your diet.

THE BODY ECOLOGY DIET

The Body Ecology Diet is probably one you've never heard of.

For one thing the diet gurus know that the Body Ecology Diet is not really as much of a diet as it is a lifelong, healthy eating plan. That by itself helps ensure people who adopt it will stick to it. In doing so, the Body Ecology Diet's creator, Donna Gates, says that you will maintain a healthier body that is less disease-prone and stronger.

Overview

The Body Ecology Diet removes sugars and the bad, saturated fats and starchy carbs from your diet. It's similar to several low-carb versions but with some twists including exercise, fermented foods, and coconut milk.

The Good...

As Dr. Joseph Mercola shows time and time again, sugar is a dangerous chemical in our bodies. Perhaps more health problems come from sugar and sources that are nothing more than disguised sugars (such as corn syrup, high fructose corn syrup, fruit juices especially those with the pulp removed, and grains and pastas that easily turn into sugar once they hit your system).

By adding healthy coconut milk (see *The Coconut Diet* for more info on that) and fermented foods such as yogurt and kefir (a type of yogurt that is said to stay in your gut longer than yogurt where it can do more good), the Body Ecology Diet takes an otherwise low-carb diet and makes it even healthier promoting long-term resistance to bacteria and infections.

The Bad and The Ugly

Hardly a downside exists with the Body Ecology Diet. Most low-carb dieters who have studied health issues from the more natural and non-pharmaceutical communities have already modified their low-carb diets to include healthy bacteria such as yogurt and kefir.

Moving to the Body Ecology Diet if you've never dieted in a similar manner might be new and difficult depending on your makeup. I suggest if that is true that you stick to it. Some people on a low carb diet, such as Neil Strauss, author of book called *The Game*, has been described as getting ill when he was told he wasn't eating enough meat at each meal. He forced himself to do that for 4 or 5 days and found that he quickly began enjoying the low-carb diet in plenty of hefty portions, far more than he ever thought possible. So don't give up.

Your Big Takeaway Tip from this Diet

The "ecology" in the Body Ecology Diet comes from the fermented foods you're supposed to eat. You are, in effect, fixing the ecology of your body, especially in your gut where so many problems can begin or be stopped with the correct flora of good bacteria that your gut needs. I love the Body Ecology Diet. Just know that some of the requirements can be strict and confusing, especially if you have never experienced making kefir or yogurt yourself.

THE BLUE ZONE DIET

"Attention! Now carb loading in the Blue Zone! The destination is where people live to be ripe old ages!"

On the planet called Earth, where do people live the longest? What cultures or regions or countries or climates seem to cultivate a long and healthy life?

Those were the questions Dan Buettner wanted answers to as he went all over the world trying to identify the aspects of diets that seemed to prolong life. The result of his globetrotting was the Blue Zones Diet.

Overview

If you eat what people eat in Okinawa, Japan and Loma Linda, California and Sardinia, Italy will you live as long as they do on the average?

Maybe the cause and effect of diet-to-lifespan is there. Or maybe we can take some of the best from each of those places and get a healthy diet from it. If so, the Blue Zones Diet is the answer because Dan Buettner took what he thought were key elements from those and other long-life areas and developed the Blue Zones Diet.

Some of the basics of the Blue Zones Diet are:

- Smaller portions

- Soy, rice, fish and a variety of vegetables

- Mediterranean dishes which are rich in grains, fruits, red wine, and short on meat

- Nuts

- Tropical fruits such as mangoes and papayas

The Good...

Smaller portions and ceasing the meal before you feel full has been shown in many studies to extend life. Perhaps it is the process of digestion that adds to our age or reduces our lifespans so smaller portions reduce our digestive requirements and hopefully adds years to our lives.

Nuts and wines and a variety of non-starchy vegetables are wonderful as long as you're not too addicted to the wine. Alcohol is based on a fermented sugar and in spite of the fact it's fermented, you don't want sugar any more than you have to.

The Bad and The Ugly

The soy is a problem, especially if you're a male who may not want to take on female characteristics. Keep soy away from the men in your life unless you stick to fermented soy products such as soy sauce and soy-based wines.

The low amounts of meat allowed in the Blue Zones Diet is certainly a problem for protein requirements. You'll be taking supplements to make up for some lost nutrients such as B vitamins if you reduce your meat intake to the levels the Blue Zones Diet requires.

The Blue Zones Diet also isn't a step-by-step, meal plan for you. You get just general guidelines, the full extent of which aren't much more detailed than what you've read here. That results in a lot of confusion and almost certainly many people adopting the Blue Zones Diet who are doing it in a manner Buettner never intended. But without specifics it's difficult to know what is exactly correct. It's also difficult to stick to.

Your Big Takeaway Tip from this Diet

The low meat portions are problematic. A doctor named Weston Price once did what Dan Buettner tried to do. Dr. Price scoured the planet looking at cultures who lived to be ripe old ages who had few health issues. The Japanese were one of the cultures he studied. And do you know what Dr. Price discovered?

Just as Buettner did, Dr. Price found several different diets in the top twelve longest-living, healthiest regions. But instead of picking what he *thought* might be contributing to the lifespan and health of each, he looked for the commonalities of all of them. The result was this: every single one of those twelve long-living cultures ate fermented foods on a regular basis. Each one ate yogurt, kefir, sauerkraut, kimchi, or fermented fish among other fermented foods.

So picking rice and soy because the Japanese people in Okinawa eat it and live a long time may have missed the boat completely. You should focus on adding to your diet fermented foods and skip trying to pick and choose from long-living cultures as diverse as the Japanese and those living in Loma Linda.

THE NEW BEVERLY HILLS DIET

Combine foods the right way and you'll be healthy and fit!

That was the goal of the Beverly Hills Diet, designed more than 30 years ago by Judy Mazel before she died at the early age of 63.

Overview

The New Beverly Hills Diet is a "new and improved" version of Mazel's original diet. Hopefully being on the new one keeps you kicking way past 63.

The New Beverly Hills Diet dictates foods that you can eat in approved combinations and not eat in prohibited combinations of foods. By putting the right foods together it is thought that you can raise your metabolism, lose weight, and stay healthier.

The rules can get complicated but here is a high-level rundown:

- You can eat proteins and fats

- You can eat carbohydrates and fats

- You can eat fruit but always by itself, never with protein, other carbohydrates, or fats

The New Beverly Hills Diet requires an initial commitment of 35 days, many of which you eat only fruit.

The Good...

Fruits are tasty so you might enjoy the New Beverly Hills Diet the first five weeks or so.

The Bad and The Ugly

Fruits are high in fructose, one of the worst sugars you can put into your body.

The New Beverly Hills Diet is complicated and not always easy to follow. In addition, you are following some rather severe calorie restrictions the first five weeks and restricting calories might be such a physical, or more likely a mental shock that you don't stick to the plan.

Your Big Takeaway Tip from this Diet

As with any calorie restrictive diet, the New Beverly Hills Diet opens you up for failure when you *really* get hungry. In addition, there is little to show that the food combinations promoted do you any good whatsoever.

THE COTTAGE CHEESE DIET

Is cottage cheese considered to be made by a "cottage industry"?

Overview

The Cottage Cheese Diet is a form of crash diet, as all of this report's diets are considered to be, and this is one of the easiest.

Given that The Cottage Cheese Diet is simple, well you know already what I'll say. That's a benefit. The easier something is to follow, the more likely we are to adhere to it.

On The Cottage Cheese Diet you do this: Eat nothing but five servings of cottage cheese and drink nothing but water for up to two weeks. If you really feel ambitious, you're allowed to put a dash of cinnamon on your cottage cheese. And for those who want to cheat, one piece of fruit with up to three of those servings is allowed.

The Good

I like cottage cheese. Scratch that, I love it!

So a diet where I eat lots of cottage cheese? Bring 'er on! The problem is, I am extremely fit, haven't gained an ounce in years, and I eat cottage cheese a lot. Still, when I see an entire diet centered around anything, even a food I love such as cottage cheese, I'm suspicious.

Let's look at it more.

The Bad and The Ugly

Again, I love cottage cheese. It is certainly a low-calorie food. In addition, it has some fermentation properties and has good protein (as long as you buy good cottage cheese).

So most exercise and weight loss gurus love the stuff and I am no exception. I've never seen problems associated with integrating cottage cheese into just about any healthy eating plan. Even Tim Ferriss who preaches, "*Never* eat any food that is white!" says cottage cheese is just fine.

But you know, none of us is going to say eating *only* cottage cheese is okay!

And after you finish your 14 days on The Cottage Cheese Diet what then?

During your Cottage Cheese Diet where are your vitamins and minerals that don't find themselves into cottage cheese and three pieces of fruit a day? Take for instance Kale, an incredible vegetable that is the most-densely packed vegetable available. Almost none of the benefits of kale come in fruit or cottage cheese!

What about essential fatty acids? What about the amazing assortment of vitamins you get in colorful veggies such as beets and squash and carrots? What about the B vitamins in grass-fed beef? What about the incredible oil and more you get with Alaskan farm-free Salmon?

You're putting yourself on the line for two weeks and demanding that your body get *none of its required nutrients* when you eat only cottage cheese and drink only water.

Ordinarily, I'd knock the three pieces of fruit aspect of The Cottage Cheese Diet (again, this is a detour from the strict originally-designed Cottage Cheese Diet that allowed only cottage cheese) for giving you way too much fructose, but with all the protein in the cottage cheese and your lack of vitamins and minerals on such a limited plan, I'd rather see you cheat with the fruit than not do it.

The fact you're told not to go past two weeks on this diet says it's not really a diet that can work long term because it's not a diet you *follow* long term.

It's for a quick bang of weight loss. And yes, it can work for two-week weight loss. And like all quick weight loss, many people go right back to their former weight and higher.

Your Big Takeaway Tip from this Diet

If you're obese, is spending two weeks to knock off the unhealthy weight worth the trade-off loss of vitamins and minerals? If you are finding no other way to get started, then dropping initial pounds for two weeks might get you started but I can assure you this: if you are currently obese due primarily because of fructose and carbs – which is why most obese people are obese – then after two weeks of having nothing but cottage cheese your chance of then taking up a healthy eating plan is the only thing that's going to be slim about you for quite a while longer.

You're far better off starting *today* eating a plan, and not a "diet," that you stick with the rest of your long and healthy-to-be life.

Skip the rope and skip the crash diets for maximum long-term healthiness and happiness!

THE PRITIKIN DIET

Nathan Pritikin developed the Pritikin Diet in the late 1970s. Several variations exist. You'll find the Pritikin Principle among others.

Overview

The Pritikin Diet recommends you eat a high-carbohydrate, low-fat, low sodium diet. Along the way you are to exercise and while you don't have to count calories there is some caloric-limiting aspects of the Pritikin Diet which are not specifically called "calorie counting."

The Good...

The Pritikin Diet's goal is to burn more calories than you take in by food. To get there you are to limit your fat intake and consume only small portions of lean meat and fish.

The Bad and The Ugly

As Gary Taubes in *Why We Get Fat* systematically proves over and over, a calorie is not a calorie when it comes to how one affects the body compared to a calorie from a different type of food.

Limiting calories to mostly carbohydrates exacerbates the problem of weight gain making every calorie that you *do* eat far more likely to stay on your hips. As I said earlier, dairy farmers feed fat-free milk to calves to *fatten the calves* and not reduce their weight. Without the fat the calves crave more carbohydrates than they otherwise would eat so they eat the corn-based grains force fed to them. This occurs in many cases because cows are built to eat grass and not grains such as corn.

Limiting your sodium intake can very well cause an electrolyte imbalance. You should always monitor your blood sodium levels if you find yourself limiting salt to make sure that you don't get too little sodium. Your body needs sodium to function properly.

Another problem with the Pritikin Diet is the exercise requirements. Yes, you'll need the exercise to help, albeit in some small way, the weight-adding carbs you're eating in bulk but the problem is this: without an ample supply or fat and protein, can you even fulfill your exercise requirements?

Your Big Takeaway Tip from this Diet

The terms "high carb" and "diet" might go well together in a sentence but those terms don't seem to go hand-in-hand in real life. Plus, the caloric restriction sets you up for failure, just as many other diets do, the moment you get hungry.

THE ACID ALKALINE DIET

Like the Hay Diet, the Acid Alkaline Diet attempts to balance your acid and alkaline levels based on the principle of pH which is a measurement of how acidic or alkaline a certain food or combination of foods are.

Eat some foods to make your blood and body more acidic and eat other foods to move them towards the alkaline side of things.

Note: Your blood's pH levels have extremely little variance in how wide of swings your blood's pH can travel from one end of the spectrum (acid) to the other (alkaline). Most pH measurements are done by your urine since your body does not have to regulate your urine's pH level as consistently as your blood's pH level.

Overview

Acid is bad!

Certainly, battery makers don't agree with that but adherents of the Acid Alkaline Diet sure think so.

They say that if your body becomes acidic, it becomes ripe for health problems. It was once said that "an alkaline body cannot get sick." (That is a loaded statement, filled with doubting Thomas's by the way.)

Supposedly our diets used to be extremely alkaline when we ate more grains and fruits and carbohydrates. This was responsible for keeping our blood pH levels intact. As modern day processing methods were invented, our foods slowly became more acidic.

The creators of the Acid Alkaline Diet say that eating meat just made that all the worse. Meat moves your body more towards an acidic state and away from the alkaline side of things.

The Good...

If your body's pH levels are greatly affected by food and if acidic pH levels do cause you health problems, then you would want to limit the foods that cause you to move closer to the acidic condition.

It might surprise you what foods produce a higher alkaline level in you. For example, lemons, while highly acidic on your tongue, change your body to a slightly more alkaline state than it was before the lemon.

Note: In spite of the fact many feel you should limit your fructose intake, lemons are wonderful additives to almost any diet. They move your pH more to the alkaline side, they reduce the glycemic damage of any food you squeeze their juice onto, and you get vitamin C and other trace nutrients too.

The Bad and The Ugly

There is little (none?) evidence to suggest that we "used to eat" grains and fruits more than we do now. The reality is that history seems to show more of a meat-eating background.

The fact that assumption might be wrong about the Acid Alkaline Diet doesn't necessarily mean the Acid Alkaline Diet is bad. But other factors might make it so. By eating a diet of grains, even if you stick to whole grains, and by reducing your meat, fish, and quality dairy products, you limit your body's ability to repair and stay healthy.

Your Big Takeaway Tip from this Diet

The Acid Alkaline Diet has been said to aid in heartburn problems over time as well as keep colds away longer than other eating plans. If you have frequent trouble with either of these problems you might want to give the Acid Alkaline

Diet a try. A warning to anyone with kidney problems is incumbent here though: the Acid Alkaline Diet can play havoc with the regular role of your kidneys.

THE 3-HOUR DIET

Popular diets seem to have the number three in their names quite a bit: the 3-Hour Diet, the 3-Day Diet...

The number 5 is popular also as in *The 5-Second Flat Belly*, and the *5-Minute Miracle Exercises*, two excellent books if I do say so myself.

Overview

Can you really lose significant weight in only three hours?

Nope! And the 3-Hour Diet doesn't make that promise.

What it does promise is to help you lose weight as long as you eat more meals in smaller portions and eat every three hours to keep your metabolism high.

The Good...

As with any portion control diet, you can eat just about any food you want on the 3-Hour Diet. Just about any kind of diet proponent will agree that multiple, smaller meals means your body will store less fat and keep its metabolism higher than would otherwise be the case with fewer large meals.

Although this is technically a portion control diet (you can't eat five large meals a day and expect any results other than possibly weighing more than you do now), the multiple meals being spaced at three hours apart from each other keeps you from becoming famished and therefore eating large quantities.

The Bad and The Ugly

The fact you *can* doesn't mean you *should* eat any food you want.

Although the 3-Hour Diet allows some cheating *once in a while*, it does also allow diet sodas which have been attributed to slower weight loss than without them. (The new soda pop named Zevia is Stevia based and contains lots of good and natural ingredients such as ginger so I'd sure suggest it over any pop whose name begins with "Diet" in its title.)

Your Big Takeaway Tip from this Diet

Even in smaller and more frequent portions, you can't go around eating whatever you like and expect to be as healthy as you otherwise would be... although in my *1 Day Diet* book (go look it up on Amazon... it's the Diet I'm most proud of) I do show you how you can eat whatever you want if you follow the program correctly.

You need to use common sense and get a variety of nutrients such as you get in quality meats, dairy, and colorful vegetables. Having said that, if you're going to help your body by eating quality meats, dairy, and colorful vegetables forget the 3-Hour Diet because portion control doesn't make any difference when you eat foods that don't add weight no matter the quantity you consume them in.

THE PERSONALITY TYPE DIET

What kind of diet needs a Psychiatrist to prescribe the food you eat?

It turns out that the Personality Type Diet doesn't. It just comes close.

Overview

The Personality Type Diet requires that you answer a series of lifestyle questions based on your preferences in food, exercise, and your ability to stick to things such as a diet.

Once you finish the lengthy set of questions, a diet is created just for you and your personality; hence, the Personality Type Diet.

The diet created just for you is mostly based on a vegetarian and fruitarian foundation with no room for high fat items. In addition, fish and chicken can be had and you can even eat red meat once in a while if you don't mind the dirty looks from the Personality Type Diet dieticians.

The Good...

In order to keep you on the Personality Type Diet, a wide variety of foods are actually allowed. But some are discouraged far more than others. Some are encouraged far more than others.

The Bad and The Ugly

The basics of any specifically-designed Personality Type Diet always seems to end up being low-fat, low-protein, high carb, and soy-based products.

You almost assuredly will need to take supplements to accent your diet.

In addition, avoid the soy no matter how much your assigned Personality Type Diet guru screams at you, especially if you're a man.

Your Big Takeaway Tip from this Diet

If you're more of a meat and dairy and fat kind of person and less of a vegetarian or (ugh!) fruitarian, you can skip the Personality Type Diet. Even though it reports to create a diet that best fits your eating and emotional preferences, what it really tries to do is fit a largely vegetarian diet to your eating and emotional preferences.

As for me and my house you can't force a square peg into a round hole. Don't design a vegetarian diet for us.

THE PERRICONE DIET

The Perricone Diet was developed by a dermatologist named Nicolas Perricone.

What a coincidence! That is almost as much of a coincidence as Lou Gehrig coming down with Lou Gehrig's disease. What were the odds?

Plus, the Perricone Diet is said to be a help as much or more for your skin as it is for your thighs and hips.

Overview

The Perricone Diet focuses on the carbohydrates you eat.

Very little distinction can be made between the Perricone Diet and several popular low-carb diets in that the Perricone Diet attempts to teach that low glycemic foods affect your weight gain the least, hence increasing your weight loss the most.

Sugar is all but banned under the Perricone Diet.

Saturated fats (the bad fats) are also eliminated.

The Good...

At first you might think banning sugar is not only a Bad and Ugly but also should be illegal but it's true that sugar causes severe healthy problems. Many health problems today, and keep in mind that your skin is the largest organ of our bodies, are attributed in part or in full to a grossly out-of-balance intake of sugar and even "natural" foods that turn to sugar rapidly such as fruit juice.

You won't be restricting calories in any way. That means hunger pangs are few and far between and perhaps will be non-existent.

The Bad and The Ugly

Very little can be said negatively about the Perricone Diet except that it does promote lean meat. As long as you eat grass-fed organic meat you don't have to worry about the fat if you prefer your beef to be marbled and tasty.

If you begin the Perricone Diet with a heavy addiction to sugar you may find yourself craving the sweets for a week or more while starting the Perricone Diet. Fortunately, the lack of emphasis on quantity means that if you get cravings you can just eat another complete meal of low-carb foods. You will soon find, as many of us have, that after a little while the sweet cravings are replaced with a much healthier yearning for some quality fish or chicken or beefsteak chased by some good colorful and leafy vegetables such as a healthy salad with real blue cheese dressing.

Nothing is said about fermented foods on the Perricone Diet. You will want to add some homemade yogurt or kefir to the Perricone Diet if you decide to adopt it.

Your Big Takeaway Tip from this Diet

The Perricone Diet is one you *can* stay on forever. The lack of sugar, the low carbohydrate focus, and the somewhat reluctant acceptance of the diet's allowance of good fats in food are focus points to consider.

Many low-carbers have been surprised to see that their skin clears up nicely with a low-carb diet such as the Perricone Diet. One might think at first that a diet which includes fats would increase the production of skin irritations such as zits but the opposite is the case. It's the sugar-based carbs that seem to damage your skin.

Note: While using your diet to fix your skin, you should also spend at least 20 minutes a day in the sun getting vitamin D3. Don't use sun screen, that stuff might cause cancer! And all that you heard about the sun itself causing cancer? Ask to see the studies! As Dr. William Campbell Douglass explains so well, there aren't any studies accurate enough to be worth reading.

THE DASH DIET

It's all about the heart!

The word Dash in the Dash Diet stands for Dietary Approaches to Stopping Hypertension.

Heart trouble is often linked to hypertension, and extreme hypertension is said to be a leading cause of death. If a diet can help the heart then that diet helps prolong life in general while it keeps away the deadly diseases related to our tickers. The Dash Diet is said to be able to reduce blood pressure for patients with problems there.

Overview

The Dash Diet mimics the FDA's Food Pyramid quite a bit. (The Food Pyramid has actually been replaced by a colorful plate of food showing recommended portions of various types of food. But most people are still only familiar with the Food Pyramid they learned about in school and saw in the papers and elsewhere our whole lives.

On the Dash Diet you are to focus on a large amount of vegetables and fruit, a slightly smaller amount of grains, and an even smaller amount of low-fat dairy and lean meats. In addition, you are to keep a check on your sodium levels.

Plus, another little thing about the Dash Diet: you have to exercise 45 minutes each day.

The Good...

Anything to help your heart, right?

The Dash Diet strongly wants you to avoid processed foods. In addition, you can move to the Dash Diet slowly and not all at once if you find it to be one you want to try but just have too much baggage from the way you eat now to move all at once.

The Bad and The Ugly

High sodium levels are certainly something to be monitored and kept in check for heart patients and potential heart patients. The problem is that sodium levels are rarely the problem by themselves. The problem as I've shown elsewhere is your sodium/potassium balance. If one or the other gets out of whack your blood pressure can be a problem.

I read and go to many types of doctors depending on what I need at the time. Much of my own doctor visits center around yearly checkups, blood tests to make sure I am regularly monitoring all my vitals, and recently I've been going through some chelation therapy to get rid of some heavy metals that seeped into my body over the years. For example, I had a high level of mercury in my blood until I replaced my mercury-laden dental amalgam fillings with inert porcelain fillings and chelated the mercury that drained from the fillings over the years out of my system.

Last year a medical doctor who did my annual checkup told me my blood pressure was too high. He wanted to put me on blood pressure medicine *that very day* which I of course refused. It's not that I didn't trust him but I'm not about to start a series of meds without a second opinion and without trying to locate the source of the trouble in my diet. Generally if you have a problem you are either not putting *in* the right things or you're not getting *rid* of enough wrong things. As I was leaving, he said, "At least start a low-sodium diet right away."

I went home that afternoon and immediately began adding large amounts of sea salt to everything I ate! (This is a true story.) And do you know what? When my blood test results from *that same doctor* came back three days later my blood showed an abnormally *low* level of sodium! If I'd followed his advice my electrolytes would be so whacky I'd be dancing the polka when I heard disco music.

60 days after increasing my salt dramatically, my blood pressure was back down to 110 over 64.

I'm taking time out of this book to tell you this story for a reason. First, you need to know *your body* better than anyone and that means better than any doctor you go to. Monitor your blood pressure, ask for a copy of every blood test you get and keep the records. Don't assume the doctor knows your body. I wasn't taking too much salt and I had actually suspected I wasn't using enough. Sure enough I was right and my blood pressure dropped like an anchor down to extremely healthy levels after two months of doing exactly the opposite of what my doctor said to do.

The Dash Diet promotes a high carb, high grain, low sodium, low-fat diet. The founders of the Dash Diet certainly have their hearts in the right place: they want you to have a healthy heart. The problem is the dramatic and massive research that shows how much *healthier* to your heart, cholesterol, and blood pressure a low-carb, high-fat (not saturated fats of course), low sugar, and basically however-much-salt-you want diet is. Dr. Al Sears constantly writes about the conclusive evidence that is found over and over showing how vapid the traditional food pyramid approach to health really is.

Don't listen just to me; instead, read all you can and make your own conclusions. But if you think the Heart and Stroke Foundation (creators of the Dash Diet) and your government are to be trusted in the face of massive research that counteracts what they promote, you might want to study some more before adopting the Dash Diet.

Your Big Takeaway Tip from this Diet

If there is anything in the food we eat that can eliminate the need for statins and other blood pressure and cholesterol and heart-related medicines, I'm in line to grab a bite!

But the Dash Diet just doesn't fly in the face of the evidence of a high-carb lifestyle. Blood pressure, cholesterol, and diabetes all seem to improve in the long run under a *low*-carb, do-the-opposite-of-the-FDA's-food-pyramid diet.

Like so many high-carb, high-grain diets, the Dash Diet requires an extensive exercise regimen of 45 minutes per day. I suspect the heavy exercise is to keep the effects of all those unhealthy grains and carbs to a minimum but one might call me cynical when it comes to such things.

THE GRAPEFRUIT DIET
(AKA, THE HOLLYWOOD DIET)

The Grapefruit Diet, aka, the Hollywood Diet, is a staple item in the diet fad industry. It's been around for about 8 decades now. That is long enough for it to come and go and come and go again for multiple generations.

You'd think if it worked it never would have gone!

Note: Yea, I'm biased against celebrity status which is why I avoid it in spite of my success at teaching others how to get fit and healthy. But I figure, if the Hollywood types were on this thing long enough for its name to be changed from Grapefruit Diet to Hollywood Diet, that is enough by itself for me to avoid it! An expert on the stage and screen doesn't make one an expert at dieting. And to look at many of today's singers and actors, it doesn't make them very slim either.

Overview

The grapefruit is sometimes called a *negative calorie food*. The thought is that in eating a grapefruit, you actually burn calories while you eat it. Whether completely true in all cases or not, that claim has some scientific basis of fact.

Several good low-carb dieting aspects are present in The Grapefruit Diet too. The diet shows some results as one would expect from a low-carb approach.

Eat a grapefruit and lose weight!

The Good

Getting thinner by eating more is certainly what we all want. If only chocolate shakes had the same properties!

On The Grapefruit Diet you are to eat one-half grapefruit at every meal. The rest of the meal is supposed to be high in fat and protein. You are to restrict all grains, starches, sugar, and non-grapefruit fruits.

The Bad and The Ugly

Fructose is the sugar found in fruits, among other more dangerous kinds of foods. Fructose is considered one of the worst carbohydrates when it comes to weight gain and other health problems.

Yes, I said it. Fruit sugar can be one of the worst sugars you ingest. I'm not alone in that assertion.

This does not mean fruit is bad – of course not! But you must watch the amount of fruit you consume. You must eat fruit that has low glycemic loads (berries are low) and you must eat the whole fruit and not just the juice. A fruit's pulp fiber reduces the damage that would otherwise be done by fruit.

Still, it doesn't take much fruit, even whole fruit, to knock your glycemic load through the roof. And if you're eating properly, meaning good animal proteins and fats and essential fatty acids, you can eat just about all the calories you want. The problem is that when you add in fructose, the fruit will work against you more and more until your daily calorie intake has nowhere to go but to your hips.

Tim Ferriss, author of *The 4-Hour Diet*, incorporates grapefruit into his eating plan one day a week but he does it *strategically*. One day a week he binges. And unlike the rumors and ripoffs of his eating plan, he systematically controls his binge day. This heavy control of his binge day, by the way, is what makes his diet *somewhat difficult to follow*. And remember, the less simplistic a plan is, the less likely we are to follow it.

One of the ways he controls his massive binging of up to 6,000 calories one day a week is to start the day with *one grapefruit squeezed into juice form* followed by coffee. Testing has shown that the *one* glass of grapefruit juice multiplies the metabolic burn of the coffee's caffeine. So drinking *one* glass of fresh-squeezed, organic grapefruit followed by a coffee chaser will prolong your metabolism's burn rate so that any cheating you do that day will be minimized to some degree.

But do you know what else Ferriss found? That doing this *more than one day a week decreased the effectiveness* of the metabolism benefit. So doing the grapefruit juice and coffee more than one day a week caused the grapefruit's fructose to kick into higher gear and hurt more than it helps!

Dr. Moreno, a dietician, states that grapefruits and grapefruit juices can interfere with prescription drugs, especially cholesterol-modifying statins. Such interaction doesn't seem to be much of a problem at low levels but "low levels of grapefruit" is not what the Grapefruit Diet promotes.

Your Big Takeaway Tip from this Diet

So what to do?

One day a week, squeeze that delicious grapefruit into a glass. Better yet, eat the whole thing and get the pulp too. And sure, if you want a grapefruit once in a while, as long as you eat the fiber and not just drink the juice, you're certainly not going to spike your glycemic much by doing so. But make it a treat and not a ritual.

THE MEDITERRANEAN DIET

I love the Mediterranean area, the Italian beaches, the slower-paced lifestyle, the wine, the long dinners, the lazy Grecian lunches, the palm trees, and everything else about it.

So, wonder what I think of the Mediterranean Diet?

The Mediterranean Diet is based on the slow-moving lifestyle of the Mediterranean area so you'd think I'd love it! (I don't hate it.)

Overview

The Mediterranean Diet is not so much a specific eating plan as it is a promotion of the Mediterranean foods.

You're encouraged to eat like the Greeks and enjoy the same long-lasting healthy lifestyles of the Mediterranean people.

To accomplish this you're to include good oils in your diet such as olive oil.

Note: always buy extra virgin olive oil and only buy it if it comes in a dark *glass* container. Olive oil spoils when exposed to light and only glass containers (not plastic!) can help ensure that the oil gets to your table in close to the same form it was shipped here in. Never use old olive oil for anything! Rancid oil affects your system in some of the same ways, albeit slower and with less impact all at once, that poison does. In spite of this precaution taking these steps to get a high quality olive oil into your kitchen is well worth the trouble.

The Mediterranean Diet also encourages you to each large amounts of fresh vegetables, nuts, fish and dairy (although in limited quantities), and even whole grains and fruits.

The Good...

As you can see from the variety of food, the Mediterranean Diet is fairly simple to stick with. You won't get bored with the food. Good olive oil is a fat that helps your skin and pleases your joints so splash it on whatever you like.

The Bad and The Ugly

Oil other than that which you find in nuts and fat from dairy products are not allowed on Mediterranean Diet. That eliminates coconut oil (surprisingly) and other oils that you might be used to using.

It turns out that meat lovers don't love the somewhat limited choice of meats on the Mediterranean Diet and Vegans don't at all want to touch the meat and dairy on the Mediterranean Diet. So while pleasing a large number of people, two other groups in general find trouble with the Mediterranean Diet to one degree or another.

Your Big Takeaway Tip from this Diet

The Mediterranean Diet is tasty and easy to follow. Your diet is fairly different from the typical American diet and you might find it difficult to eat out most places and still adhere to the Mediterranean Diet. Still, if you're willing to cut back a bit on the recommended grains, I think you'll have good results with it.

THE ZONE DIET

The Zone Diet isn't as much of a diet as it is a complete universe!

Books and products galore have been written, created, designed, and sold that center around and promote the Zone Diet.

Created by the now-wealthy Dr. Barry Sears, his Zone Diet is easily one of the most popular diets of the past 100 years. Although it has slightly fallen out of favor in recent times, many Zone products still sell and many people still go on the Zone Diet – and are *still* on it – after many years.

Overview

The idea of the Zone Diet is to get into the zone. Literally!

The Zone Diet's premise is that certain food combinations put us in a zone where weight loss occurs more easily and naturally. Also, our yearning for more and more food is satisfied and our bodies adapt to a smoother eating pattern that is easier to maintain than our typical grab whatever we see or want is.

The bottom line is that to get into this "zone," men can eat 14 blocks of food and women can eat 11 daily. Different foods have different block values. Once you hit your block maximum, you're done eating for the say.

The Good...

If hunger is your downfall, get into the zone. Proponents of the Zone Diet say that hunger and cravings are a thing of the past when they reach the zone.

The Bad and The Ugly

The Zone Diet is quite complex actually in spite of the harmless-sounding block approach. Trying to figure out how many blocks of food are in front of you and keeping tabs on how many blocks you've eaten so far for the day is daunting. Many of the Zone Diet products and books try to take away some of that confusion.

Your Big Takeaway Tip from this Diet

A simple diet is one more people will follow. The Zone Diet is complex and not simple. If you're good with rules you'll be fine with the Zone Diet and may like staying on it a long time. Eventually, people get "fed up" with the counting of the blocks. Fortunately, by then many of them have developed sort of a sixth sense as to what they can and cannot eat while still remaining on the Zone Diet so that isn't always the problem it sounds to be at first. Still, there are far simpler diets that are as effective or more so.

THE NEGATIVE CALORIE DIET

The Negative Calorie Diet says that the more you eat the more weight you lose.

This conjures memories of the *Grapefruit Diet* we studied earlier and many of the same principles apply here.

Overview

You might recall that digestion is one of the highest energy-consumption function your body can perform. Yes, you do lose weight by digesting your food. The question is this: is there food that takes *so* much energy to digest that the mere digestion of it makes you weigh less after it's gone through your mouth and stomach than before?

The Negative Calorie Diet says yes and that foods such as grapefruit (of course), pineapples, oranges, apples, and more are negative calorie foods that burn more weight than they add.

Be careful though and read the Negative Calorie proponent's carefully. Not all fruits and vegetables are negative calorie foods so you can't be a happy Vegan.

Turns out you can't be a happy meat eater either.

The Good...

No grains are promoted on the Negative Calorie Diet so you don't get the negative effects of corn or cereals. In addition, you avoid possible gluten allergies since bread is out of the picture.

The Bad and The Ugly

Where's the beef?!

The Negative Calorie Diet allows no room for meats or nuts or essential oils. You have to consume a massive amount of supplements if you go on the Negative Calorie Diet to meet your daily minimum requirement of even some basic nutrients.

Your Big Takeaway Tip from this Diet

Just say no to Negative Calorie Diet. It is as bad as much as it sounds good.

THE ABS DIET

Our final diet focuses on something every lady (and man) wants whether we admit it publicly or not: great, sexy abs!

Overview

The goal of the Abs Diet is to remove fat from our bellies primarily. While we've been taught that spot losing isn't possible, Tim Ferriss offered some interesting and different possible conclusions in the *4-Hour Body* and the creators of the Abs Diet say their eating plan *can* attack the belly fat.

While not specifically a diet, the Abs Diet comes in two flavors: one for men and one for women. While similar you will get the best results by choosing the one for you obviously.

You must eat breakfast and you should exercise with this plan. You can't add sugar to anything. Of course those aspects of the Abs Diet are good to follow with any healthy eating plan.

You then can choose from twelve foods to eat from at mealtime:

- Almonds and nuts

- Beans

- Spinach and green, leafy veggies

- Dairy

- Instant oatmeal

- Eggs

- Turkey and lean meats

- Peanut butter, but it needs to be as organic and natural as possible and not *Jif* no matter how good that stuff tastes!

- Olive oil (see my note about olive oil in <u>The Mediterranean Diet</u>)

- Whole grain bread and cereal

- Extra protein powder in whey form

- Raspberries and strawberries and blueberries and blackberries

Notice the first letter of these twelve foods spell out *Abs Diet Power*.

Yea, it's kind of a gimmick but there are far worse food choices in some of the other diets!

The Good...

The variety of the Abs Diet is nice.

That variety makes it easier to stick with and enjoy.

The Bad and The Ugly

The dairy is to be non-fat. I'll bet you a nickel that if you ignore that requirement and drink raw, whole milk you will lose *more* fat than you would if you believed the lie that skim milk makes you skinnier.

In addition, don't worry so much about your meats being lean. Worry more that they are organic, or locally-grown and grass-fed (being grass-fed is more important than being organic).

Also, trade the instant oatmeal, if you must eat the grains once in a while, with some freshly-flaked oat groats (oatmeal in its unpressed state) to ensure you get vitamins that are present in fresh-flaked oatmeal that doesn't make it to your pantry through normal grocery story channels.

Note: Why did the creators of the Abs Diet put *instant* oatmeal on the list? I think it's because they needed an *I* in that position!

Your Big Takeaway Tip from this Diet

Men especially can get health maladies with a tire around their middle. And women love to show off their thin waists to men (and to other women but we will never admit we are so showy when we've got it to show!).

If the premise is true that the Abs Diet attacks our middles and puts our bellies back to beautiful, then there is little to find that's not to like. I'd cut back a bit on the grains (actually, I'd eliminate them but I'm extreme) and up the fat in the dairy and meat but other than minor tweaking, the Abs Diet is simple to follow and is varied enough to keep you on it without getting tired of it too soon.

QUICK LOOK DIET TIPS CHEAT SHEET

Below are all fifty *Big Takeaway Tips* that appear at the end of each of this book's diets. This quick-reference list gives you a handy rundown and summary of the good, the bad, and the ugly with each one.

The 17-Day Diet

Variety is the spice of life and being on a diet that changes its food contents every 17 days has appeal. To many people, especially women, eating the same basic diet for long term can get monotonous. Men typically can do better on the same food for longer periods of time but everybody can get tired of the same old food.

So for variety, the 17-Day Diet is one you probably won't become bored with.

In addition, if the premise that rapid weight loss is better than slow weight loss – which again goes against the grain of every diet plan ever studied – then if true, you can find other diets that take off more with less effort. You can even try one of the starvation diets and have more rapid weight loss than the 17-Day Diet provides. (I am not recommending any starvation diet.)

Note: I'm just saying you could lose more weight faster. The problem is you'll almost certainly put it right back on and more after you finish the starvation diet.

The 17-Day Diet is better for your health than a starvation diet even if it's not as rapid in its weight loss.

The China Study Diet

There is absolutely *no way* that a vegan diet can be the reason the Asians showed less disease over the more meat-intensive West if the meat- and animal-fat-only Inuits also showed a lack of such diseases when they ate virtually no vegetables whatsoever their entire lives.

Instead of focusing on the actual foods you eat, you should focus on the *source of those foods*. No study has ever shown that raw milk is bad for you or that grass-fed beef is bad for you or that mercury-free wild Alaskan salmon is bad for you. Quite the opposite.

If you hate the taste of meat, don't eat meat. But if you like meat make sure you eat well-sourced meat that you know the origins of. Enjoy that steak, or heck, enjoy as much seal blubber as you like, as long as you know the animal was not pen-raised with hormones and antibiotics given from birth and fed nothing but corn.

The Sonoma Diet

Given that carbs equal bigger thighs, any food variety that includes them requires that you eat in moderation. When it comes to starchy and virtually fiberless carbs (such as corn, potatoes, rice) you need to reduce your intake of those dramatically to see a prolonged weight loss and you need to stay off those foods to keep the weight off.

Given that it's the reduction in these carb quantities that probably contribute the most to the Sonoma Diet, you might want to short-circuit the time required to lose weight and skip the Sonoma Diet and focus on one that concentrates more fully on eliminating the bad carbs altogether.

Still, if you're hungry and find yourself needing a change for a while, not dramatic weight loss, the Sonoma diet is not a horrible diet to be on and its restrictions, while not offering rapid weight loss, do provide weight loss eventually. And slow and steady weight loss is certainly the rate most agree is best for a good, long-term healthy weight.

Eat Right for Your Type / The Blood Type Diet

Given the problems of the Blood Type Diet, why not avoid it and find a more sensible solution if possible?

The Carbohydrate Addict's Diet

The basis for the Carbohydrate Addict's Diet is sound: eating protein-rich foods and healthy oils while curbing the carbs is a proven way to lose weight in a healthy manner. So many more low-carb diets, however, while being stricter than the Carbohydrate Addict's Diet, certainly are better recipes for weight loss at a more reasonable speed (meaning faster than the Carbohydrate Addict's Diet but not too fast).

Biggest Loser Club

As with any calorie-limitation diet, the Biggest Loser Club sets up many for failure as soon as hunger pains kick in... and hunger pains *always* kick in. The variety of this diet, including the use of grains, causes it somewhat to be a fat-producing eating plan. The limit on the calories works only because you're actually being limited on the carbs you eat.

The exercise portion of the Biggest Loser Club will help you get toned and turn some flesh into muscle but in general the food you eat impacts your weight far more than any exercise you do.

No Sugar, No Flour

As with any calorie-limitation diet, the No Sugar, No Flour Diet will show weight loss but is also prone to cause you to stumble later when your full feeling doesn't last as long as it should.

The South Beach Diet

Once you get to your ideal weight, you can monitor the South Beach Diet and stay on the diet for life if you'd like. The variety of foods might make that possible. The carbs allowed in the second phase doesn't make the South Beach Diet as rapid of a weight loss diet as many low-carb diets can do but it's thought that if you lose weight slowly but surely you are more likely to keep it off and notice the effects of the diet less.

Rosedale Diet

The lack of balance of the Rosedale Diet causes it to have problems and failures. Still, if you find yourself in an extreme state that requires an instant pouncing of your hunger, losing your first several pounds on the Rosedale Diet might be what you need to get started. Its complete lack of grains and carbs, especially for the first few weeks, keeps those danger foods away which will help you move to a more protein-rich diet after you've found success on the Rosedale Diet.

Weight Loss Cure

Stay away from any "diet" that promotes hormone injections!

If your doctor tells you that you need such injections for any reason, first get a second opinion! If they both agree, then you may need to follow their advice or better yet, get new doctors. But don't volunteer for those.

With so many other options available, stay away from the Weight Loss Cure until further notice!

The Oatmeal Diet

If you insist on eating grains and increasing your fiber, you could do worse than oatmeal. (For example, you could eat corn!)

But before grabbing that big tub of oats or (worse!) a packet of instant oats, consider buying a bucket of organic *oat groats*. You can get these at Walton Feed (http://www.waltonfeed.com). Next, get you a flaker which is an attachment for a meal grinder and grind a fresh cup of oats before you eat them. This way you get the nutritional benefits of oatmeal. The nutrient loss of oatmeal after it's been flaked already is rapid. By the time it gets packed in containers and shipped to your local store, the oatmeal still has its fiber but hardly any nutrition.

Better yet, enjoy your fresh-ground oatmeal as a treat once in a while instead of making it your primary source of food by going on the Oatmeal Diet. That way you don't get so many problems from the heavy-grain and carb diet and you can enjoy a *nutritious* bowl of oatmeal as a treat every once in a while.

The Rice Diet

If you have kidney or hypertension problems by all means give the Rice Diet a try. You will probably lose some weight and hopefully you'll lose the health problems.

If that happens you may want to then switch to an eating plan that you can stick to for life.

The Cabbage Soup Diet

My prescription for you? Eat that cabbage soup as often as you want, at any meal you want, any day you want, and try to get some fermented cabbage in the form of sauerkraut several times a week too. You'll get fantastic nutrients and good bacteria in your gut as well.

And as a bonus, the bulk in the cabbage might be good to help you feel more full... so by having a pre-entrée cabbage soup you might skip the post-entrée dessert!

Bottom line? Don't skip the cabbage or the cabbage soup... skip the Cabbage Soup Diet.

Pocket Diet

Portion control is important if you want to eat virtually anything you want. Why add to your body's caloric and grain burden however by eating everything inside pita bread? Skip the pita bread and you free up a few more calories that you can make up with something else you really wanted. You won't get the heavy grain hit if you skip the pita pockets too.

In addition, the six-week limitation of the Pocket Diet means that you must change your eating plan once you finish the Pocket Diet. Any "diet" that is not truly a long-term eating plan sets you up for failure when you "end" the diet. Look for something that you can actually live with for the long term. Anything else deserves the name "fad diet."

The Japanese Diet

If you can manage portion controls *and* eat only healthy, fresh, unprocessed, in-season foods, you'll get no argument from me about the Japanese Diet's possibilities. Smaller portions, perhaps several times each day makes sense because gobbling a large meal all at once is shown to put on more poundage than spreading the same number of calories across time or meals on the same day.

P90X Nutrition Plan

Only the most dedicated stay with the P90X Nutrition Plan for long.

You will see results early due to the complete lack of bad carbs in the first few weeks. This weight will be real weight loss and not just water loss. In addition, the exercise will work to get your muscles and toning agents working overtime.

If sticking-to-it isn't your middle name, however, you might find other diet plans easier to stick with. In addition, as I've said elsewhere in this book, any diet plan that ends after a fixed amount of time means that it's not an eating plan for life. Mentally, having a stop date for any diet might – and often does – encourage you to unconsciously develop a back-to-normal eating style once the diet ends. And normal is what might have gotten you into this mess in the first place!

The O2 Diet

In spite of its adherence to high ORAC foods, the O2 Diet is little more than a low-fat, high grain, high fruit, and high vegetable diet. You and your family's bodies were designed to eat protein, especially animal protein and fats. There are some wonderful antioxidant-rich supplements on the market. The best might just be astaxanthin. Take it daily and skip the low-fat diet that has been shown to be a colossal failure in almost every form it's been tried for the past 80 years.

Naturally Thin Diet

I worry about your protein levels if you stick to the letter of the law on Naturally Thin. Finding a general eating plan that includes lots of strength-retaining and damage-repairing animal protein, while limiting grains, fruits, and fiberless starchy carbohydrates through portion control ensures your body gets more of what it needs while you still limit portions of the bad foods. In addition, the not-bad foods such as grass-fed beef and wild Alaskan salmon you can eat *as much as you want* so you won't even know you're on portion-control rationing if your diet is a good one. That's a plan you can stick to forever.

The Banana Diet

The devil is in the details of *any* diet. With The Banana Diet you must drink room temperature water with the banana. And "anything else you want to eat" is quickly censored by the diet's designers when they warn you can have no dessert after your evening meal, you can't eat after 8pm, and you must be asleep by midnight.

All of which is good advice on any diet and by themselves those three limitations should help reduce weight – all things being equal – for any eating plan.

Oops. Two more things. No more dairy or alcohol. Processed dairy certainly has problems but if you have a local farm nearby who supplies you with delicious dairy products (especially with healthy whole, raw milk) then you've just eliminated a major source of energy and nutrients from your diet. And not having even a small, single glass of wine has drawbacks both socially and, yes, even for your health in the long-term if you'd otherwise have a little wine.

Maker's Diet

As you can see and as one would expect, the Maker's Diet focuses far more heavily on the physical aspect of the diet than the promised mental, emotional, and spiritual aspects. Still, the detoxification foods, the suggested supplements, and the overall approach of becoming more aware of potential problems that may be active in your body and soul, is not a bad recipe for a healthy lifestyle.

Ketogenic Diet

I like the Ketogenic Diet. I'd modify it from two days of high carbs down to just one. One is enough to keep your leptin in check. In addition, I warn you strongly against 5 days of aerobic exercises each week. Not only do *most* find that level of activity unsustainable (thereby quitting all exercise) but new research is screaming at us describing the benefits of interval aerobics.

Look into some of what Dr. Al Sears, M.D., has developed with the PACE program. This basically involves exercising for as little as *10 minutes* to get the same results as 30-to-45 minutes of high-intensity aerobics. His PACE program and others like it suggest you do low-heart rate exercise such as walking for 2-3 minutes followed by high-intensity power-walking or even running if your body can take it for a minute or so. Then alternate this 3-minute walking with 1-minute high-heart rate aerobic exercise for 4 or 5 times. The result is a far greater fat loss than seen otherwise.

Dr. John Ratey, M.D. describes near the end of his book *Spark* that this kind of interval exercise was the only way he could lose the last few pounds of fat from around a man's trouble area: the belly.

Hungry Girl Diet

There's nothing wrong with looking at Hungry Girl Diet recipes to get some good food preparation tips. You will find ways to avoid calories that otherwise might enter your stomach. Be cautious that you don't overdo artificial sweeteners (better yet, avoid them altogether or use Stevia) and lowering animal or real dairy fat too much can work against your weight as much as it can work for you.

No S Diet

Overall, the No S Diet gets a grade of A from me. As you may have gleaned from this book, I think research tends to favor a low-carb diet as one that is easiest to stick to and lose weight on but I think the No S Diet will work for many people who have failed at lots of other diet attempts in the past.

Fat Loss 4 Idiots

Don't be an idiot! Avoid the Fat Loss 4 Idiots Diet!

Actually, there are far worse diets out there, many are described in this book. But in general a low-fat diet, especially one that is scheduled to end after so many days, will probably give you short-term weight loss at the expense of not enjoying yourself during the process and returning to your previous ways of weight gain afterwards.

Eat to Live

Whenever you eat, whatever you choose, wherever you go, always increase the benefit of your food by eating as healthy of ingredients as possible. Opt for raw vegetables over cooked. Opt for medium or even rare beef over well done. If you must eat bread, do the work and grind organic wheat into flour right before you bake your own bread. That kind of bread has lots of benefits in spite of the carbs but be sure and butter it liberally with homemade, organic butter to slowdown the glycemic impact.

Other than the healthy ingredients, the Eat to Live Diet doesn't offer a lot of long-term success promise. It's like so many other low-fat, heavy vegetarian diets.

The Diet Solution Diet

I don't know the percentages of people who fall in the different types but it's my suspicion most people are typed as protein and a protein/carb mix type. While promoting healthy organic and unprocessed ingredients as much as possible while warning against soy, the Diet Solution Program has little I can find that is a problem.

The hGC Diet

Keep in mind the hGC Diet was introduced in the 1950s so we have decades of studies about it.

And according to Dr. Oz, a man with whom I don't always agree with, it's difficult to argue that over a dozen trials have been made, all centered around the hGC Diet, often replacing the hGC with a salt-fluid injected placebo, and the resulting weight loss numbers were *no better* than using the expensive, side-effect potential, costly hGC hormone injection.

The Coconut Diet

I really like the foundations of the Coconut Diet and I rarely like any diet that focuses heavily on one specific food. Having said that, I promote the theory that a diet that is simple to follow is one that *will* be followed. The Coconut Diet isn't simple. If you decide not to adopt the Coconut Diet, I'd still suggest you find some of that delicious, organic, extra-virgin coconut oil and use it in as much food preparation as you are able.

Fruitarian Diet

The biggest benefit to the environment you might make if you adopt a pure Fruitarian Diet is the large number of bacterial elements in the soil that your early-to-grave body provides the bugs and crawly things as your coffin disintegrates six feet under. Just avoid this diet or I'll go "bananas!"

The Hay Diet

Did Dr. Hay get better because of his diet or did he get better *while* trying his diet? Clinical studies have not shown the Hay Diet to be extremely reliable.

The Ornish Diet

Gary Taubes in his *why We Get Fat* book shows study after study and clinical trial results right and left showing the weight-loss and major health benefits of animal proteins and good fats and oils. It appears that Dr. Ornish disagrees with the doctors that Taubes cites considerably. If you're a vegetarian you probably will do better under the Ornish Diet than the Fruitarian Diet.

French Women Don't Get Fat

If you fail at diets that are extra strict and if you like yogurt (I don't like it but I eat it daily; you should too!), you might do very well the rest of your life living like the Mademoiselles live so give the French Women Don't Get Fat Diet a try.

Eat Clean Diet

If portion control has been a problem before, you may really like the Eat Clean Diet. You can basically eat as much of the legal foods as you wish and probably still lose weight. You should follow the yogurt suggestion to get your probiotics although staying away from processed foods is a great step towards keeping your stomach's good bacteria. The Eat Clean Diet stresses a little too much leanness for my taste – lean meat, egg whites only, etc., which has been show to slow down instead of ramping up weight loss but in general if you can maintain a natural food lifestyle you will enjoy the Eat Clean Diet.

The Baby Food Diet

Keep in mind, a big advantage of baby food is that it is said not to be processed as much as other foods can be. (You'd better make sure of these claims for your baby's sake by the way. Making your own is always best.) In addition, baby food doesn't have as much sugar or additives as the processed foods we can buy. You can even get gluten-free baby food if you have a problem with allergies or think you might have a problem with allergies.

But every one of those benefits is true of any and all healthy food that you should be eating.

By limiting yourself to baby food, you are paying far more for the same food you'd get elsewhere in larger quantities. The only advantage is it comes in little jars you can use later for make-up I suppose!

Real food – it's what your teeth were designed for.

The Chocolate Diet

If you're truly having a chocolate problem, the Chocolate Diet can turn you from a raging chocoholic into a slightly slender, less raging chocoholic. The chance that this diet will cure us of this wondrous devilish delight is slimmer than you and my waists cut down halfway. It is said that dark chocolate provides some health benefits in the form of some fermentation-like properties. (Too bad because I prefer the milk chocolate.) So if you must cheat, see if the dark stuff can satisfy you.

Once your cravings are reduced from the Chocolate Diet consider going on a lifelong eating plan that does not count calories or remove a lot of fats from your diet.

Body Ecology Diet

The "ecology" in the Body Ecology Diet comes from the fermented foods you're supposed to eat. You are, in effect, fixing the ecology of your body, especially in your gut where so many problems can begin or be stopped with the correct flora of good bacteria that your gut needs. I love the Body Ecology Diet. Just know that some of the requirements can be strict and confusing, especially if you have never experienced making kefir or yogurt yourself.

Blue Zones

The low meat portions are problematic. A doctor named Weston Price once did what Dan Buettner tried to do. Dr. Price scoured the planet looking at cultures who lived to be ripe old ages who had few health issues. The Japanese were one of the cultures he studied. And do you know what Dr. Price discovered?

Just as Buettner did, Dr. Price found several different diets in the top twelve longest-living, healthiest regions. But instead of picking what he *thought* might be contributing to the lifespan and health of each, he looked for the commonalities of all of them. The result was this: every single one of those twelve long-living cultures ate fermented foods on a regular basis. Each one ate yogurt, kefir, sauerkraut, kimchi, or fermented fish among other fermented foods.

So picking rice and soy because the Japanese people in Okinawa eat it and live a long time may have missed the boat completely. You should focus on adding to your diet fermented foods and skip trying to pick and choose from long-living cultures as diverse as the Japanese and those living in Loma Linda.

New Beverly Hills Diet

As with any calorie restrictive diet, the New Beverly Hills Diet opens you up for failure when you *really* get hungry. In addition, there is little to show that the food combinations promoted do you any good whatsoever.

The Cottage Cheese Diet

If you're obese, is spending two weeks to knock off the unhealthy weight worth the trade-off loss of vitamins and minerals? If you are finding no other way to get started, then dropping initial pounds for two weeks might get you started but I can assure you this: if you are currently obese due primarily because of fructose and carbs – which is why most obese people are obese – then after two weeks of having nothing but cottage cheese your chance of then taking up a healthy eating plan is the only thing that's going to be slim about you for quite a while longer.

You're far better off starting *today* eating a plan, and not a "diet," that you stick with the rest of your long and healthy-to-be life.

Skip the rope and skip the crash diets for maximum long-term healthiness and happiness!

Pritikin Diet

The terms "high carb" and "diet" might go well together in a sentence but those terms don't seem to go hand-in-hand in real life. Plus, the caloric restriction sets you up for failure, just as many other diets do, the moment you get hungry.

Acid Alkaline Diet

The Acid Alkaline Diet has been said to aid in heartburn problems over time as well as keep colds away longer than other eating plans. If you have frequent trouble with either of these problems you might want to give the Acid Alkaline Diet a try. A warning to anyone with kidney problems is incumbent here though: the Acid Alkaline Diet can play havoc with the regular role of your kidneys.

3-Hour Diet

Even in smaller and more frequent portions, you can't go around eating whatever you like and expect to be as healthy as you otherwise would be. You need to use common sense and get a variety of nutrients such as you get in quality meats, dairy, and colorful vegetables. Having said that, if you're going to help your body by eating quality meats, dairy, and colorful vegetables forget the 3-Hour Diet because portion control doesn't make any difference when you eat foods that don't add weight no matter the quantity you consume them in.

Personality Type Diet

If you're more of a meat and dairy and fat kind of person and less of a vegetarian or (ugh!) fruitarian, you can skip the Personality Type Diet. Even though it reports to create a diet that best fits your eating and emotional preferences, what it really tries to do is fit a largely vegetarian diet to your eating and emotional preferences.

As for me and my house you can't force a square peg into a round hole. Don't design a vegetarian diet for us.

Perricone Diet

The Perricone Diet is one you *can* stay on forever. The lack of sugar, the low carbohydrate focus, and the somewhat reluctant acceptance of the diet's allowance of good fats in food are focus points to consider.

Many low-carbers have been surprised to see that their skin clears up nicely with a low-carb diet such as the Perricone Diet. One might think at first that a diet which includes fats would increase the production of skin irritations such as zits but the opposite is the case. It's the sugar-based carbs that seem to damage your skin.

Note: While using your diet to fix your skin, you should also spend at least 20 minutes a day in the sun getting vitamin D3. Don't use sun screen, that stuff might cause cancer! And all that you heard about the sun itself causing cancer? Ask to see the studies! As Dr. William Campbell Douglass explains so well, there aren't any studies accurate enough to be worth reading.

Dash Diet

If there is anything in the food we eat that can eliminate the need for statins and other blood pressure and cholesterol and heart-related medicines, I'm in line to grab a bite!

But the Dash Diet just doesn't fly in the face of the evidence of a high-carb lifestyle. Blood pressure, cholesterol, and diabetes all seem to improve in the long run under a *low*-carb, do-the-opposite-of-the-FDA's-food-pyramid diet.

Like so many high-carb, high-grain diets, the Dash Diet requires an extensive exercise regimen of 45 minutes per day. I suspect the heavy exercise is to keep the effects of all those unhealthy grains and carbs to a minimum but one might call me cynical when it comes to such things.

The Grapefruit Diet – Hollywood Diet

So what to do?

One day a week, squeeze that delicious grapefruit into a glass. Better yet, eat the whole thing and get the pulp too. And sure, if you want a grapefruit once in a while, as long as you eat the fiber and not just drink the juice, you're certainly not going to spike your glycemic much by doing so. But make it a treat and not a ritual.

Mediterranean Diet

The Mediterranean Diet is tasty and easy to follow. Your diet is fairly different from the typical American diet and you might find it difficult to eat out most places and still adhere to the Mediterranean Diet. Still, if you're willing to cut back a bit on the recommended grains, I think you'll have good results with it.

The Zone Diet

A simple diet is one more people will follow. The Zone Diet is complex and not simple. If you're good with rules you'll be fine with the Zone Diet and may like staying on it a long time. Eventually, people get "fed up" with the counting of the blocks. Fortunately, by then many of them have developed sort of a sixth sense as to what they can and cannot eat while still remaining on the Zone Diet so that isn't always the problem it sounds to be at first. Still, there are far simpler diets that are as effective or more so.

Negative Calorie Diet

Just say no to Negative Calorie Diet. It is as bad as much as it sounds good.

Abs Diet

Men especially can get health maladies with a tire around their middle. And women love to show off their thin waists to men (and to other women but we will never admit we are so showy when we've got it to show!).

If the premise is true that the Abs Diet attacks our middles and puts our bellies back to beautiful, then there is little to find that's not to like. I'd cut back a bit on the grains (actually, I'd eliminate them but I'm extreme) and up the fat in the dairy and meat but other than minor tweaking, the Abs Diet is simple to follow and is varied enough to keep you on it without getting tired of it too soon.

SUMMARY

So there you have it. Those are fifty different crash diets for women (and men) that I hope you think long and hard before you consider doing any of them.

Some are great and some are not. All have *some* basis in truth of course or they would never have been adopted past the first few failures. If you can read between the lines, there are some things you can take from some of those diets that can be useful and helpful to add to your own diet plan.

If you're truly interested in a long term healthy diet for weight loss that makes sense and isn't hard to do, I urge you to check out my book called *The Ultimate Diet Guide*.

It's pretty much the easiest diet you could ever go on. And many dieters consider my **1 Day Diet** book even better if you want faster results.

I hope you enjoyed this book and you found it helpful in regards to what diets to avoid completely while also picking up some tips and ideas on what you can incorporate into your own diet.

As a free bonus for reading this book, please look below about how you can get another one of my books for free. This book sells for $19.95 elsewhere, but I want you to have it for free.

Sincerely,

Jennifer Jolan

Here's A FREE Gift Just For Trying This Book Out

America's #1 Weight Loss Queen Reveals How to Lose an Entire Dress Size In 2 Weeks Or Less Simply By Spinning Around In A Circle... Like a 4-Year Old Child...

"Over 120,000 people have read my book and it normally sells for $19.95 elsewhere, but you can have it for free and in your email box in just 5 minutes by going to the link below!" - Jennifer Jolan

To Claim Your *Free* Book

http://WeightLossEBookStore.com/bonus

Here's what you'll learn inside:

- The scientific reason why spinning in a circle produces rapid weight loss (if you do it the right way).

- The correct direction to spin in for maximum results.

- The exact speed to spin if you want to burn the most weight. (And exactly how often you should do it!)

- How to supercharge your energy levels and literally "de-age" your body by spinning around the right way.

- The reason why spinning will balance out your hormones. (Unbalanced hormones could very well be the ONLY reason why you're overweight -- here's how to get them in balance fast!)

- Why spinning the right way can keep you thinner and living longer than everyone around you. (Even if you live the same lifestyle they do!)

- What you should do with your TV when spinning to ensure the most weight loss in the quickest time.

- And much, much more.

This book contains one of the most fascinating weight loss methods you'll ever use.

There's no hard exercise necessary.

And no restrictive dieting needed.

Just spin around the way Jennifer Jolan describes and watch the pounds fall off faster than you ever thought possible.

To Claim Your *Free* Book, Go To:

http://WeightLossEBookStore.com/bonus

COPYRIGHT AND TRADEMARK NOTICES

products and services) mentioned in this book should be performed or otherwise used without clearance from your physician or health care provider. There may be risks associated with participating in activities or using products mentioned in this book for people in poor health or with pre-existing physical or mental health conditions.

Because these risks exist, you will not use such products or participate in such activities if you are in poor health or have a pre-existing mental or physical condition. If you choose to participate in these risks, you do so of your own free will and accord, knowingly and voluntarily assuming all risks associated with such activities. The materials in this book are provided "as is" and without warranties of any kind either express or implied. The Author disclaims all warranties, express or implied, including, but not limited to, implied warranties of merchantability and fitness for a particular purpose. The Author does not warrant that defects will be corrected, or that that the site or the server that makes this book available are free of viruses or other harmful components. The Author does not warrant or make any representations regarding the use or the results of the use of the materials in this book in terms of their correctness, accuracy, reliability, or otherwise. Applicable law may not allow the exclusion of implied warranties, so the above exclusion may not apply to you.

Under no circumstances, including, but not limited to, negligence, shall the Author be liable for any special or consequential damages that result from the use of, or the inability to use this book, even if the Author or his authorized representative has been advised of the possibility of such damages. Applicable law may not allow the limitation or exclusion of liability or incidental or consequential damages, so the above limitation or exclusion may not apply to you. In no event shall the Author's total liability to you for all damages, losses, and causes of action (whether in contract, tort, including but not limited to, negligence or otherwise) exceed the amount paid by you, if any, for this book. You agree to hold the Author of this book, the Author's owners, agents, affiliates, and employees harmless from any and all liability for all claims for damages due to injuries, including attorney fees and costs, incurred by you or caused to third parties by you, arising out of the products, services, and activities discussed in this book, excepting only claims for gross negligence or intentional tort.

You agree that any and all claims for gross negligence or intentional tort shall be settled solely by confidential binding arbitration per the American Arbitration Association's commercial arbitration rules. All arbitration must occur in the municipality where the Author's principal place of business is located. Arbitration fees and costs shall be split equally, and you are solely responsible for your own lawyer fees. Facts and information are believed to be accurate at the time they were placed in this book. All data provided in this book is to be used for information purposes only. The information contained within is not intended to provide specific physical or mental health advice, or any other advice whatsoever, for any individual or company and should not be relied upon in that regard. The services described are only offered in jurisdictions where they may be legally offered. Information provided is not all-inclusive, and is limited to information that is made available and such information should not be relied upon as all-inclusive or accurate. For more information about this policy, please contact the

Author at the e-mail address listed in the Copyright Notice for this book.

IF YOU DO NOT AGREE WITH THESE TERMS AND EXPRESS CONDITIONS, DO NOT READ THIS BOOK. YOUR USE OF THIS BOOK, PRODUCTS, SERVICES, AND ANY PARTICIPATION IN ACTIVITIES MENTIONED ON THIS BOOK, MEAN THAT YOU ARE AGREEING TO BE LEGALLY BOUND BY THESE TERMS.

Made in the USA
Lexington, KY
30 June 2012